total
tai chi

total tai chi

matthew rochford

expert consultant peter warr

THUNDER BAY
P·R·E·S·S

San Diego, California

Thanks and acknowledgments to:

Ali, Peter Warr, Andrew Broadhead, Chris Waters, Stephen Wakely, my family, all students past and present at TTP, all students past and present of the Devon School of Tai Chi, all students past and present on the Wu Kung TTP, Lavinia Soo-Warr, Karen, Ljiljana and Kate at MQP, Mark, Mike and Mark at the photo studio

Thunder Bay Press
An imprint of the Advantage Publishers Group
5880 Oberlin Drive, San Diego, CA 92121-4794
www.thunderbaybooks.com

SERIES EDITORS: Kate John, Karen Ball MQ Publications
EDITORIAL DIRECTOR: Ljiljana Baird, MQ Publications
PHOTOGRAPHY BY Mike Prior
DESIGN BY Balley Design Associates

ISBN 1-57145-934-0
Library of Congress Cataloging-in-Publication Data available upon request.

Printed in China
1 2 3 4 5 07 06 05 04 03

contents

introduction to tai chi

Tai chi is a unique activity that bridges the gap between ancient and contemporary. There are more people practicing it today than at any other time, though to many Western minds it still seems to be something rather foreign and strange. But the beauty and peacefulness of tai chi is clear to all observers. The movements embody qualities we react strongly to: calm, fluidity, correctness. Tai chi represents some important human and philosophical principles, such as relaxed power, wisdom in action, ancient knowledge, respect for tradition, and being a peaceful warrior.

Attractive in form, tai chi is also a very useful and practical art. For millions of people, it gives a distinct advantage in life, as all the benefits detailed in this book will show. Tai chi practice is one of the best ways to combat stress, ill health, and aging while keeping your body fit and flexible. The life skills learned while accruing knowledge of the art are invaluable: patience, determination, mental focus, and the ability to affect one's health positively are things we can all benefit from.

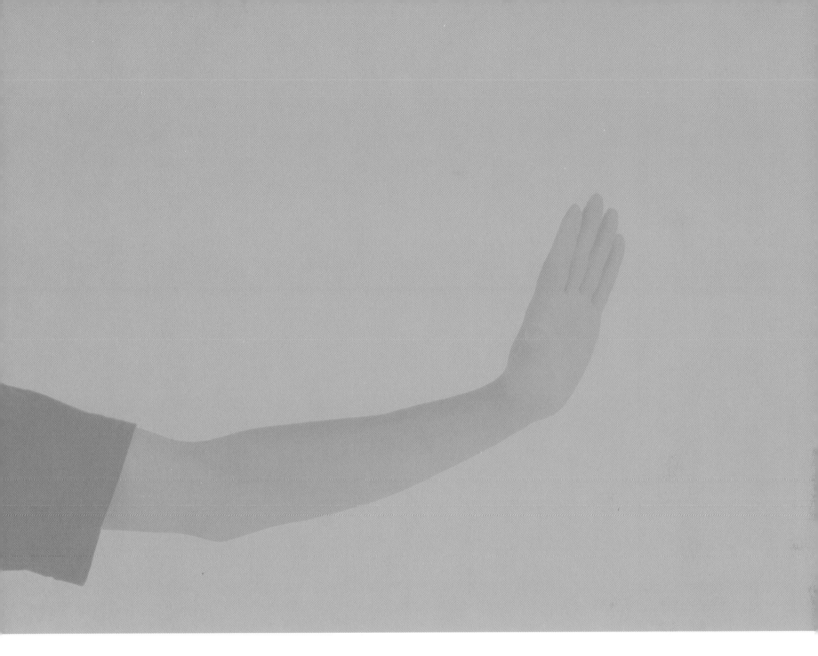

Learning such an activity from a book undoubtedly presents challenges to both the reader and the writer. However, this book will give you a very clear and easy-to-follow set of exercises that you can begin to benefit from in a very short space of time. I have tried to make the progression within the book as logical as possible and have used the help of my teacher, Peter Warr. We believe this book will provide an excellent introduction to tai chi and a crucial learning resource throughout your tai chi journey from beginner to experienced practitioner.

Whatever your reason for reading this book, be it as an introduction, an enhancement to your existing knowledge, or as a source for teachers themselves, we welcome any feedback and questions that you can send to us via the contact information in the back. If you have any medical conditions that you think may be affected adversely by the exercises in this book, please check with your physician prior to trying them. The exercises in this book, however, are all safe and will present little or no risk to the vast majority of people. Enjoy!

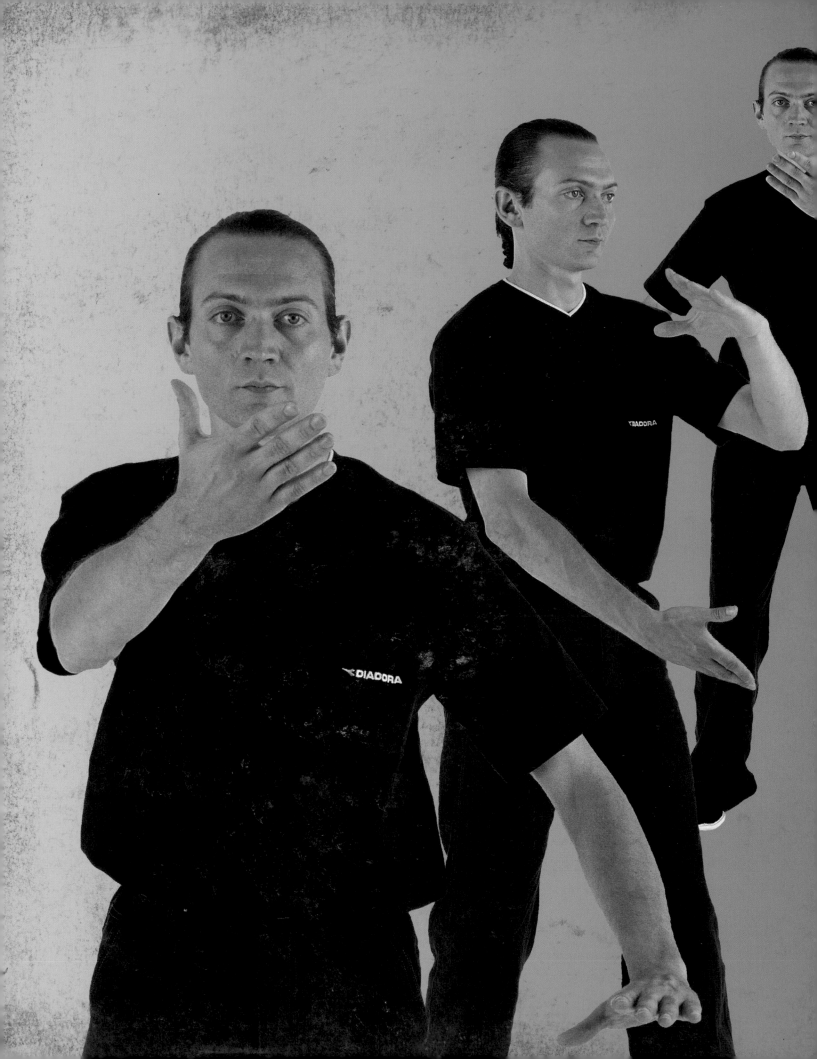

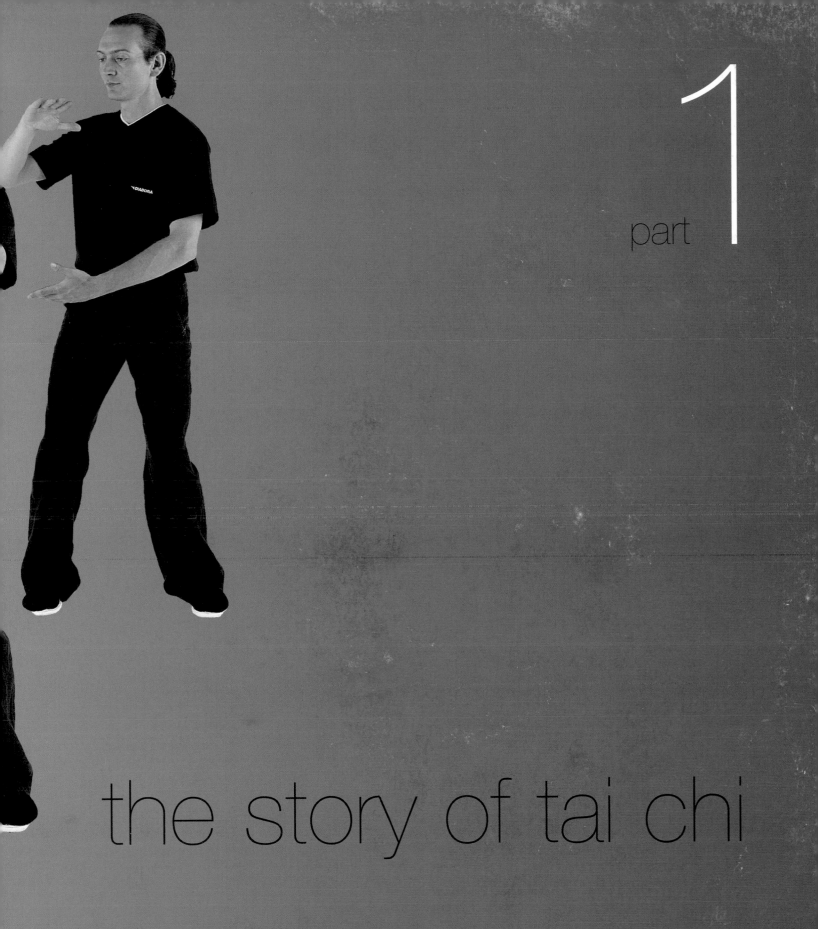

the story of tai chi

an ancient martial art

an ancient martial art and form of moving meditative practice

Tai chi is becoming increasingly well known as a way of reducing stress and improving peace of mind and spiritual well-being. Known as an internal art because of its emphasis on energy cultivation and meditation, tai chi has become very popular, largely because it counteracts the effects of stress, aging, and illness. Tai chi also allows the practitioner to protect himself or herself from attack through its highly effective martial applications. Tai chi is often referred to as "shadow boxing" because its gentle, sequential movements can be compared to a slow martial arts routine with an imaginary partner.

left: The calligraphy character representing *chi*

Many people who have seen tai chi practiced in parks or on television recognize it as a slow, dancelike form of movements with similarities to martial arts. However, in its fullness, tai chi encompasses both self-defense and the development of the mind. The benefits of practice are immense and can offer something to most, if not all, people in the world today.

As an activity, tai chi can leave you breathless with its grace and beauty and surprise you with its power and precision, but many people do not realize that if they practiced a little every day, their health and well-being would improve significantly.

Tai chi was first mentioned in the *I Ching* (The Book of Changes), an ancient Taoist oracle and book of wisdom that was written between 3000–1100 B.C. Literally translated, *tai chi* means "supreme ultimate reality" or "essential forces that govern all phenomenon." In the symbolism of Taoist philosophy, tai chi is represented by Yin, the passive, absorbing force that is considered feminine, and Yang, the active, penetrating force that is considered masculine. Yin and Yang emerge from the void (Tao) to interact and create all things that exist. This is the basis of all phenomena in Taoism, one of China's three major religions/philosophies.

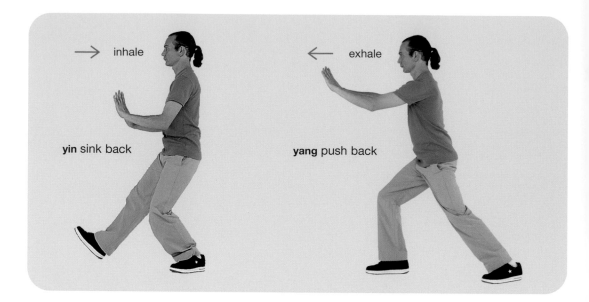

inhale →   yin sink back

← exhale   yang push back

Storing energy is like drawing a bow;
    releasing energy is like shooting an arrow.

Tai Chi Classics

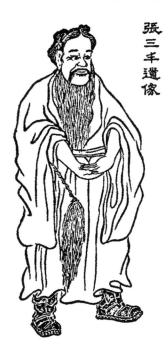

above: According to Chinese folk legend, Chan Sang Feng was the inventor of tai chi.

the history of tai chi

Tai chi is a popular form of exercise today, but the origins of this art lie in medieval China, where matters of life and death relied upon martial art skills.

According to Chinese folklore, the creator of tai chi chuan was a Taoist sage named Chan Sang Feng, who lived in the thirteenth century. According to the many legends associated with him, he traveled extensively throughout China, eventually settling at the Wu Dang Mountain, famous for the spiritual practices of Taoism and for Wu Dang Kung Fu (a version of kung fu used in the film *Crouching Tiger, Hidden Dragon*). Apparently, the inspiration for tai chi came when he watched a fight between a snake and a crane—noting not only the graceful movement of each creature, but also the way in which each creature held its own. Although it seems likely that someone called Chan Sang Feng did exist, there is little historical evidence to confirm that he was the creator of tai chi chuan as we know it today.

Exercises similar to tai chi and Chi Kung likely existed in China for thousands of years. Archaeological information suggests that such activities were present from the

Chou Dynasty (1100–221 B.C.). Chinese history is rich with philosophical teachings and spiritual practices and has a well-documented culture influenced by Buddhism, Taoism, folk religion, militarism, and Confucianism. It was against this backdrop that tai chi emerged and rose to become one of the most revered martial arts in China.

Deciphering tai chi history is far from easy, and almost every source of information on the subject differs. However, tai chi does have a common ancestry and connections with Chan Sang Feng (real or imaginary) and, more verifiably, with the Chen family and their village in the Hebei province. It was in the Chen village that the term "tai chi chuan" was first used and where martial arts fused with Taoist alchemy and military strategy to produce this unique art.

below: Lao Tzu founded the philosophy that inspired tai chi.

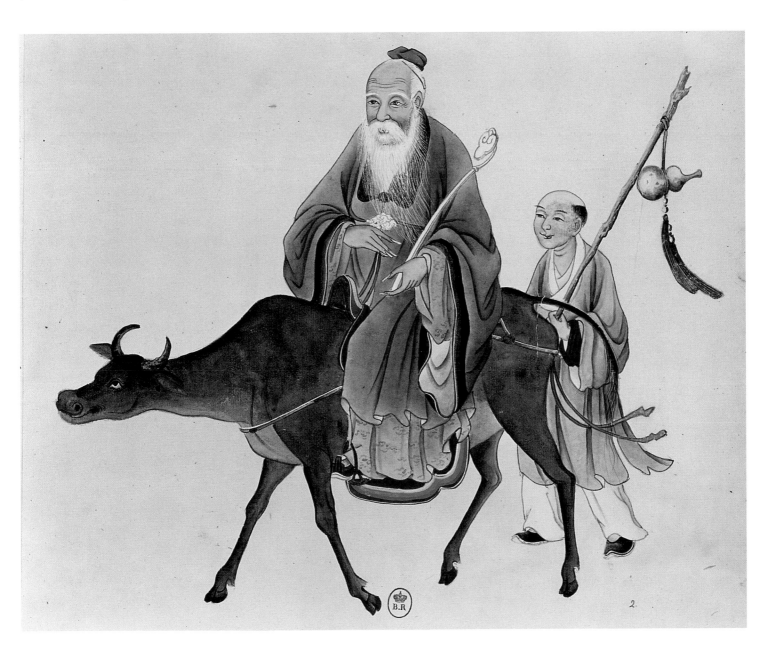

The Chen family can trace their art back to the sixteenth or seventeenth century, and writings on tai chi chuan started to appear at the end of the nineteenth century. The first written text specifically on tai chi chuan was written by Wang Zong Yue and was entitled *Tai Ji Quan Lun: A Discourse on Tai Chi Chuan.* For many years the Chen family kept their art secret and nobody outside the clan was allowed to learn the system. The reasons for this were, first, that their art was very useful, and second, that their village's security relied on it. Any leakage of technique or information was an extremely serious matter. This remained the case until Yang Lu Chan (the father of the "Yang style") learned the art after secretly observing the family training sessions while working as a servant in their house. When discovered, Lu Chan had to pit his skills against the family—and won. He was then accepted into the family and developed his art to a very high level of skill, earning the nickname "Yang the Invincible."

After Yang Lu Chan's acceptance into the Chen family, he took tai chi chuan to his home in Yongnian and then later to Beijing, exposing the art to the outside world for the first time. The secrecy that surrounded tai chi wasn't just broken by Yang Lu Chan alone: The cultural climate of China was changing, especially after 1900 and the failed Boxers' Rebellion. After the martial artists failed to remove the Japanese and Europeans from Beijing, the cultural perspective of martial artists as invincible was brought down to earth. The gun and bullet were now seen as what they were—sadly, more effective than hands and swords. It was during the twentieth century that tai chi became a practice more oriented toward health and less toward martial skill. Although the true masters of the art were still great fighters, the general population after 1956 were offered tai chi as a health system (in simplified forms developed in Beijing by Professor Li Tien Ji, for example). Although the Maoists destroyed so much, they eventually fostered tai chi as a way of maintaining the country's health, which meant that tai chi survived as an activity and involved millions of people. The "Beijing forms" of the practice are still being developed today and have their place within the world of tai chi. They provide logical and clear progressions, high levels of practitioner excellence, and aesthetic and athletic development.

From the 1800s, tai chi developed into many versions and several distinct styles, all of which connect back to the Chen style. The Chen style contains different versions, as does the Yang style. Each generation added their own influence and this process of development has given us a rich and diverse art form. From the Yang and Chen styles, the Wu (Hao) style emerged. From the Yang style, the Wu (Woo) style was created. From a fusion of the Wu (Hao) style tai chi and two other internal martial arts, Ba Gua and Hsing I, came the Sun style. Each style has its own substyles and there are styles with different lineages in the same family.

tai chi family tree

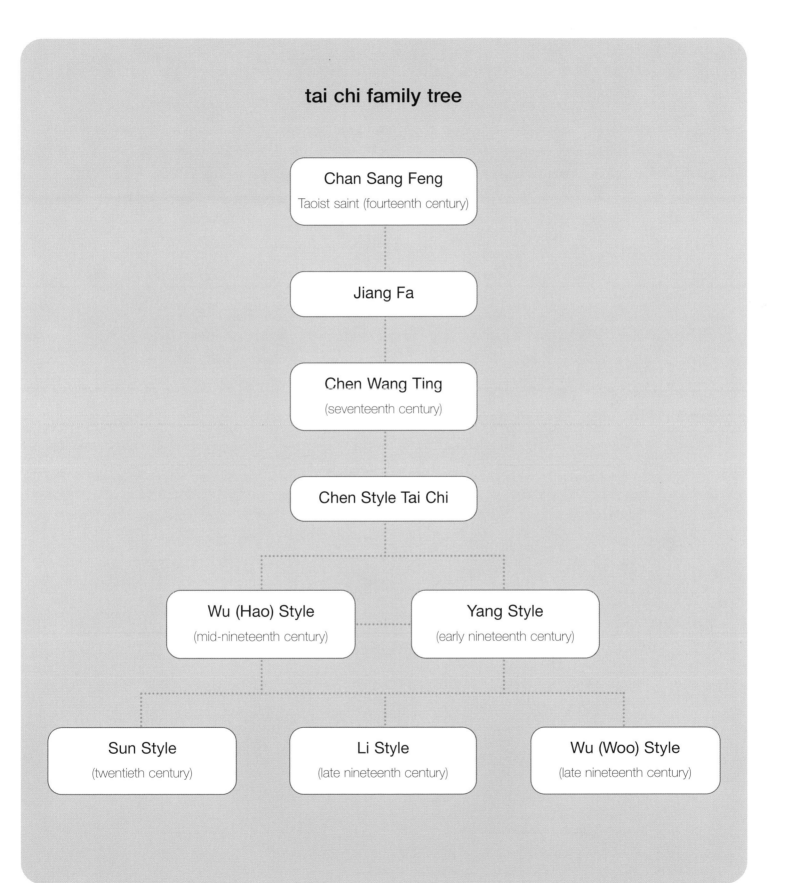

Chan Sang Feng
Taoist saint (fourteenth century)

Jiang Fa

Chen Wang Ting
(seventeenth century)

Chen Style Tai Chi

Wu (Hao) Style
(mid-nineteenth century)

Yang Style
(early nineteenth century)

Sun Style
(twentieth century)

Li Style
(late nineteenth century)

Wu (Woo) Style
(late nineteenth century)

different tai chi styles

While all the styles of tai chi share the same philosophical framework and many of the essential points for practice are the same, the outer appearances, even within a style, can be very different. This reflects how tai chi has been adapted to suit different people, times, and uses. Throughout its many generations, tai chi has often evolved and changed. The various styles of tai chi include:

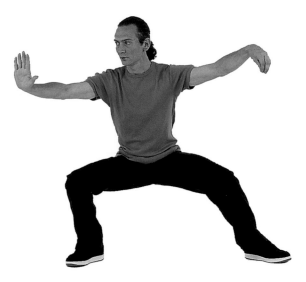

single whip stance, chen style

the chen style
- Many low, physically demanding stances
- Obviously circular and spiraling movements
- Slow, flowing movements
- Fast, explosive movements
- Overtly martial in appearance
- Very long and, more recently, short forms
- Slapping and kicking movements

As the original tai chi, the Chen style is the most demanding to learn. The physical demands of the Chen style are perhaps not for the fainthearted, but in recent years shorter, more basic versions have been introduced to make it more accessible.

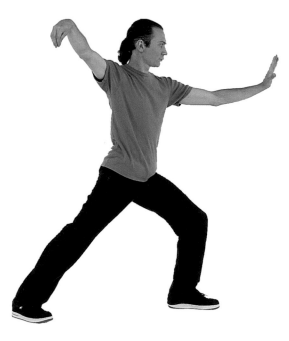

single whip stance, traditional yang style

the yang style
- Larger movements
- More covert, spiraling movements
- Slow, evenly-paced forms
- Covertly martial
- Long and various short forms

This is the most widely practiced style of tai chi.

The Chen style evolved into the Yang style during the nineteenth century via Yang Lu Chan. His sons also practiced their father's art and his grandson Yang Cheng Fu is credited with being the father of modern tai chi.

The Yang style is characterized by large, flowing movements, with little emphasis on fast or explosive movements. The martial power of the Yang style is covert, hidden within its intricate, large, circular movements. Yang style today is mainly practiced for health, although it is still being studied as a martial art in its fullness by a minority of practitioners. Within this style there are many versions, depending on the lineage. Roughly speaking, Yang style can be divided into:

• The traditional forms (although there is more than one version, depending on the lineage).
• Modern simplified forms (mainly developed in Beijing; for example, the 24-posture sequence or the form illustrated in this book).
• Cheng Man Ching style (developed in the 1950s by Professor Cheng Man Ching).

These are the main Yang style variations, but the characteristics are generally the same depending on lineage. Cheng Man Ching's version, for example, is characterized by softer, more compact movements than other versions.

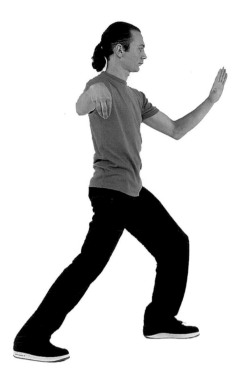

single whip stance, cheng man ching style

the wu (woo) style
• Medium-sized movements
• Long, medium, and, more recently, short forms

Sometimes known as Woo (Manchu) style, the Wu (Woo) style is derived from the Yang style of Yang Ban Hou. The Wu (Woo) style was created by Wu Chuan You in the latter part of the nineteenth century. The original form consisted of eighty-five movements, but a form with fifty-seven movements also exists. It is characterized by smaller movements than the Yang style, but larger movements than the Hao style.

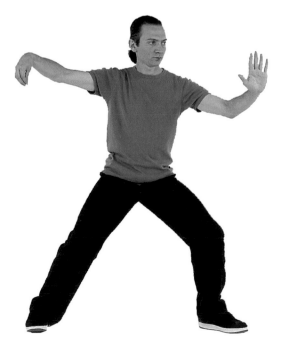

single whip stance, wu style

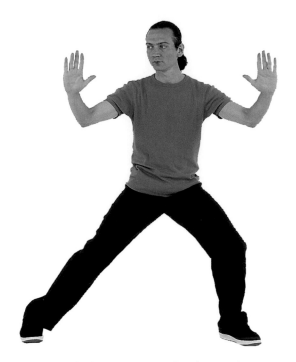

single whip stance, hao/sun style

the wu (hao) style

• Small, circlular movements
• Very simple and uncomplicated external movements

The Wu (Hao) style is derived from the small-frame style of Wu Yuxiang and is one of the lesser-known styles of tai chi. Characterized by minimal external movement and maximum internal focus, the moves of the Wu (Hao) style are not much to look at when compared to the Yang or Chen styles. However, the style is equally effective and as powerful as any other style, both for health and self-defense. Grand Master Liu Ji Shun, who lives in the U.S., is the current lineage holder of this style and there are relatively few practitioners but, perhaps, a uniquely pure lineage. The Wu (Hao) style is characterized by obvious opening and closing movements (as seen in its derivative, the Sun style). The stances are relatively high and narrow, making it quite easy to learn from a physical point of view.

the sun style

• High stances
• Obvious opening and closing movements
• Aspects of Bagua and Hsing I Chuan merged with tai chi
• The most recent, distinct style

Sun Lu Tang, a leading tai chi master, developed this style after many years of martial arts study. Known as the "Living Monkey King" because of his incredible martial skill, Sun Lu Tang was a master of tai chi and two other internal martial arts, Bagua and Hsing I Chuan. The Sun style is characterized by small, nimble movements.

the li (lee) style

• Small and medium-sized movements
• Shares features of Wu (Woo) and Wu (Hao) styles
• Exact origins still being researched

The Li style is something of a mystery, and its true origins are still uncertain. One line of thought is that it came from Li Yi Yu (1852–92), a Hao style master, but this has not been established. A famous teacher, Chee Soo, popularized the Li style between the 1960s and 1980s, and it is still taught today. Lavinia Soo-Warr is the main lineage holder of this style.

below: It is popular practice to perform tai chi out in the open air.

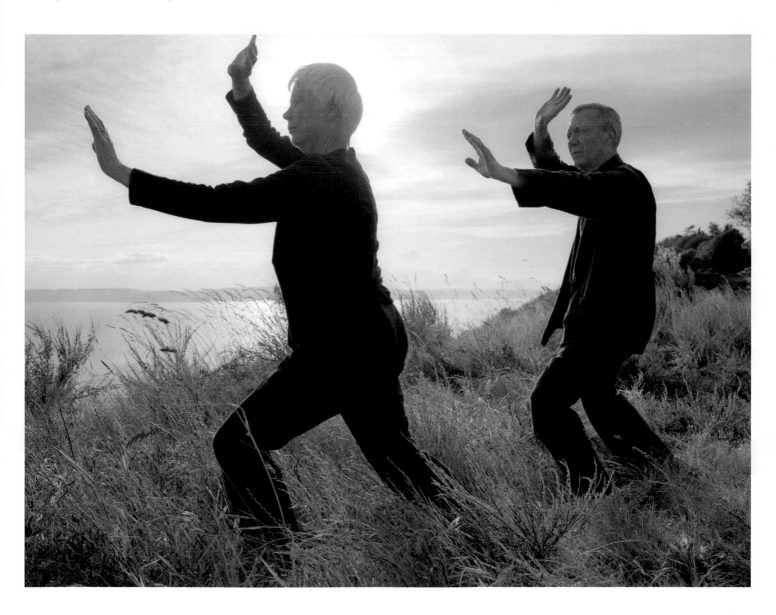

tai chi and twenty-first-century life

So being and nonbeing produce each other:
Difficulty and ease complement each other,
Long and short shape each other,
High and low contrast with each other,
Voice and echoes conform to each other.
Before and after go along with each other.

Tao Te Ching, Verse 2, "Everyone Knows"

The essence of tai chi is harmony and balance. If we go out of balance, we need to find it again to reestablish our well-being. Tai chi is rebalancing. It complements the fast pace of life we lead and contrasts with the "must have now" tendency of our age.

Tai chi has always evolved and today we see a huge proliferation of styles, masters, and routines, both traditional and modern. Tai chi has grown tremendously in popularity over the last decade and now almost every town and city has tai chi classes. One of the most enriching aspects of tai chi is its ability to grow and change into a more relevant system of development for today's world. The late Master Huang Jifu said during a seminar some years ago: "You must be flexible in your life." He meant that tai chi is not separate from life and should never become institutionalized. The issue for modern tai chi is to resolve the conflict between what is appropriate for the age and what is traditional.

One of the main reasons many people attend classes is to escape the stresses caused by our modern lifestyles. The pressures of daily life are perhaps more noticeably stressful now than they have ever been. The technological advances of the last century have changed our world forever, providing most of us with a high standard of living and even higher levels of convenience. However, the resources needed to create this state have placed us, and our planet, at risk. As we strive to be successful, make a living, and realize our potential both vocationally and financially, the tendency to work long hours has become the norm. The effect of this is to create a lack within us—physically, emotionally, and spiritually. It is this lack that tai chi can help us with through the practice of its unique movements and principles.

In Taoism, any extreme cannot last long and inevitably changes into its opposite. If I were to overwork every day and maintain high-intensity activities in my free time, it would be not be surprising if I eventually became run-down. If I continued to work and play hard, driven by the desire to succeed at all costs and continued using up any reserves of energy within my body because I was unwilling to listen to the messages it was giving me, I would become ill. This pattern of goal-driven behavior illustrates that an extreme of activity and overwork (Yang) is not sustainable and will inevitably lead to an extreme of inactivity (Yin) while I recover my energy. It is patterns like these that are behind many of today's ailments: burnout, migraine headaches, heart problems, mental exhaustion, and in extreme cases, emotional breakdown.

Success and prosperity, material happiness, and abundance are all worthwhile goals, but when the desire to achieve these things drives us to extremes, we need to try a different path.

The tai chi symbol is about balance and the practice of tai chi is also about balance: restoring balance and harmony to our lives. As an activity, tai chi helps us forget about the concerns of the day and allows us to turn inward; we focus on our breathing, posture, movement, and our mind-body connection.

Unlike virtually any other form of activity, tai chi is slow—the antithesis of modern life. Tai chi dissolves tension and pain caused by stress, anger, and overwork, leaving us feeling refreshed through the performance of the soft, flowing movements and

below: Tai chi is a form of exercise that can be praticed by young and old alike.

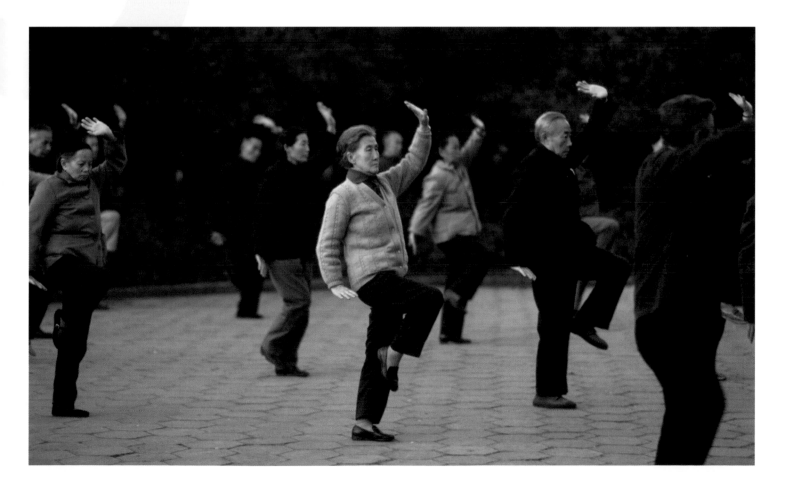

rejuvenated by its strength and power. In time, these effects intensify, but you can feel the benefits from just one session. Though as with learning anything else, tai chi requires a certain amount of perseverance in order to reap the full benefits.

The effect of doing something so slowly, in a relaxed way, can calm the nervous system down after a hectic day, or if you have been feeling "down," it will bring your body to life again. The gentle movements of tai chi cause a muscular action similar to massage, which, in turn, stimulates the lymphatic system, cleansing the blood of toxins, boosting the immune system, and heightening your sense of physical well-being. The meditative effects include mental calm and an improved ability to concentrate. Breathing is also enhanced by practicing techniques that focus on breathing with the diaphragm. Another benefit of diaphragmatic breathing is that lung elasticity has been shown to improve. Tai chi may also help lower blood pressure.

Many fitness activities improve your fitness levels but can leave your system exhausted and your joints aching. Although activities such as aerobics, running, and weight training are beneficial in moderation, they are unlikely to leave you feeling calm and peaceful, and if practiced too vigorously, they can cause damage to the muscles, joints, and the heart. Many athletes are plagued by injury and minor illnesses such as colds and flu, but by practicing tai chi as a warm-up they can decrease the risk of injury and boost their immune system.

below: Tai chi classes are now very popular in the Western world as an antidote to high-stress lifestyles.

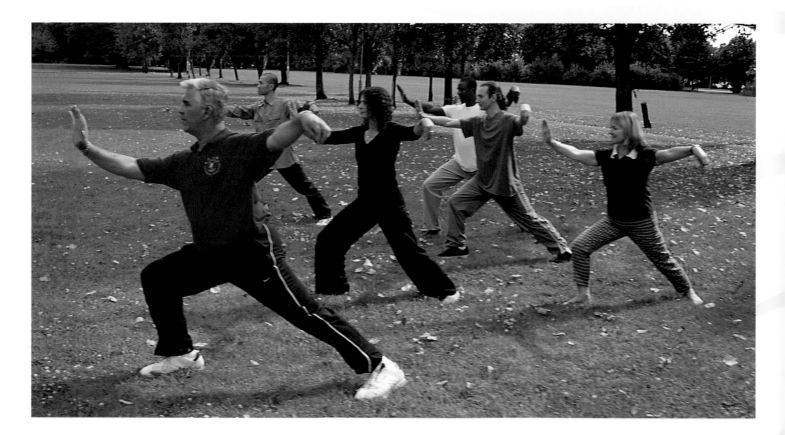

tai chi and you

> ## Nothing in the world is more flexible and yielding than water
>
> *Tao Te Ching*, Verse 78, "The Most Flexible Thing in the World"

Tai chi is a bit like water, the softest and most flexible of elements. The essential qualities of tai chi are derived from its unique set of principles, which, throughout the different styles of tai chi, include:

- **Postural guidelines**
- **Mental intent and calm**
- **Raising the spirit**
- **Breathing (physical and energetic aspects)**
- **Use of waist to direct movement**
- **Turning on the central axis of the body**

In terms of an holistic therapy, tai chi works on your mind, your body, your energy, and your spirit. It is this unique and practical synergy that makes tai chi so effective.

Of course, what you get from tai chi depends on a range of factors. For example, if you train a lot and learn advanced forms and martial techniques, you will become much fitter and will build up your stamina and internal power, providing you can find a good teacher. If you are older, perhaps what you want is more relaxation, flexibility, and balance. Consequently, the benefits will be different.

One of the strongest features of tai chi is that the qualities and benefits of practice are not limited just to the times when you exercise. The practice of tai chi can, and does, have several added benefits. Something peaceful and good for your body is nourishing to the soul, and just the achievement of finishing a form will boost your confidence and self-worth. Many of my novice students think it will be too difficult to do tai chi, having seen the complex moves performed in class. In reality, I have never taught anyone who was not able to learn the movements and underlying principles. The only quality they needed is persistence, applying it to the goal in a patient, determined way.

Often the problem, whether it be practicing tai chi or a life dilemma, is in our own minds; thinking in a positive way usually helps. It is similar in combat: You cannot rely on what you have been told—you must think and decide for yourself and respond in the moment, otherwise you will be caught off-guard. The warrior is part of us all and through understanding tai chi we can become better equipped to overcome problems and seek positive outcomes.

One of the most famous tai chi masters, Yang Lu Chan, was known as "Yang the Invincible." Legend has it that although he defeated many other martial arts masters, he never hurt any of them. This story illustrates two things: first, that tai chi is very effective as a martial art, and second, that positive outcomes can be found even in the most difficult of situations. The positive outcome of this warrior's fighting skill was that no one was hurt, which is a huge achievement.

below: The flexibility and power of water, as highlighted in the *Tao Te Ching*, can be compared to tai chi.

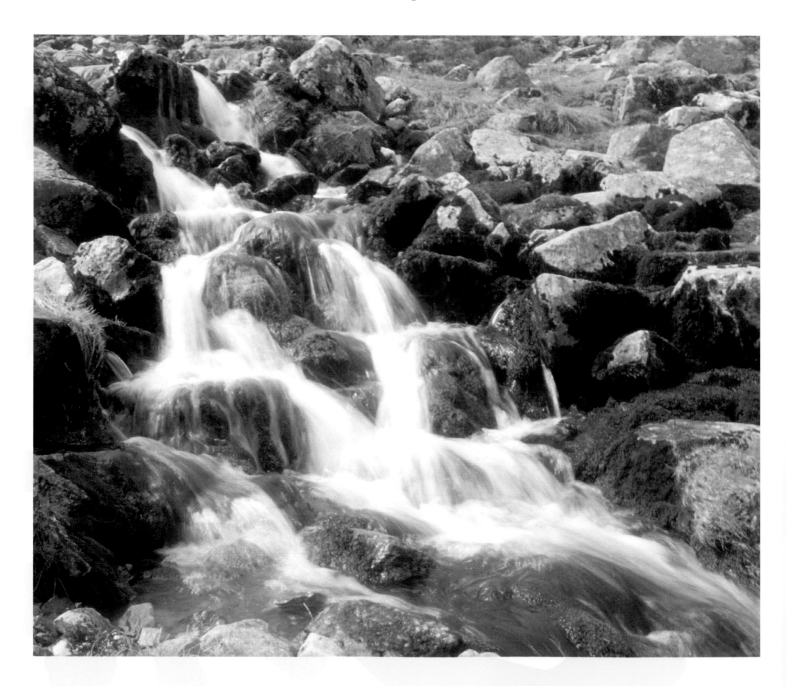

physical benefits

The movements of tai chi work on many levels, both obvious and hidden. First, the posture of tai chi improves general well-being and attitude. Second, the internal organs begin to function more effectively as they are aligned and positioned correctly. Third, the gentle movements softly massage the internal organs, further boosting their effectiveness, blood and energy supply, and strengthening the connective tissues between them. This also keeps the internal organs from becoming too damp (a condition recognized by Chinese medicine), which can lead to many ailments.

Muscularly, the whole body is worked with tai chi. Leg muscles become stronger, back muscles are strengthened through the seated posture of tai chi, the muscular system of the body is toned and balanced throughout via the equal workout you do on both sides of the body. Recent medical research has pointed to the following health benefits associated with tai chi practice:

- Blood pressure is more balanced
- Less fatigue
- Less likelihood of falls (for the elderly)
- Increased white blood cell count (for the immune system)
- Increased breathing capacity
- Improved postural control
- Improved heart health in older people

Exponents of tai chi claim that tai chi was good for migraines, asthma, arthritic and rheumatoid conditions, back and postural problems, insomnia, psychological problems, injury recovery, and recovery from many illnesses.

Several factors affect our body's ability to function well:
- Our ability to relax
- Our posture and body alignment
- Our breathing

One of the most important principles within tai chi is relaxation (or *song* in Chinese). Without this alert but relaxed and strong emphasis in tai chi, our *chi*, or life-giving energy, is impeded and blocked, and the fluidity of movement cannot occur. When we move in a relaxed but confident manner, we save energy and we flow. Relaxation is not a state of collapse, but rather a sense of being present in the body; alert but not tense and fearful. Thus the body language of a tai chi practitioner is not aggressive or passive; it is in the middle of these two extremes.

Some of the benefits of tai chi for the body include:

• Improved digestion and circulation via gentle abdominal massage during the waist-directed movements
• Improved blood circulation via the gentle stimulation of the movements
• Improved organ function due to correct posture and organ position
• Lymphatic drainage via the muscular stimulation of that system
• Greater oxygenation of the blood via improved breathing
• Improved brain function due to more oxygenated blood circulating
• Improved flexibility in the joints by means of increased synovial fluids
• Core stability muscles in the back are strengthened
• Buildup of tension in the shoulders is addressed and reduced
• Prevention of conditions such as osteoporosis, rheumatoid arthritis, and low or high blood pressure
• Improvement of many physical conditions, including back problems
• Significant leg strengthening and muscle toning
• Improved performance for athletes

While working with elderly tai chi students, I have noticed that they have more focus and concentration; those with chronic illnesses have more energy and a greater sense of well-being; people with back problems improve dramatically; those with poor balance due to inner ear problems experience an improvement. Overall, I would say that tai chi has the potential to benefit anyone's health.

modern life	tai chi
fast paced	slow and carefully paced
time pressures	time to unwind and refocus
worries about the future	being in the present moment
competitive	noncompetitive
stress	de-stressing
emotionally draining	rejuvenating
risk of burnout	recharging batteries
culture of consumerism	there is nothing to buy—just practice
"I want it now"	developing patience

tai chi and energy cultivation

One of the aims of tai chi practice is to cultivate chi (energy) at the lower Tan Tien—a center of energy believed to be located just below the navel. This "inner alchemy" is part of the ancient Taoist path to longevity and, ultimately, immortality.

The basic idea here is that where the mind goes, the energy follows—something that is also used in the martial side of tai chi. When one focuses the attention at the lower Tan Tien, the tendency is for chi to gather there and a feeling of well-being to ensue. You feel very centered after doing this for several minutes. The lower Tan Tien is the very center of the body and is the main center of energy that controls vitality,

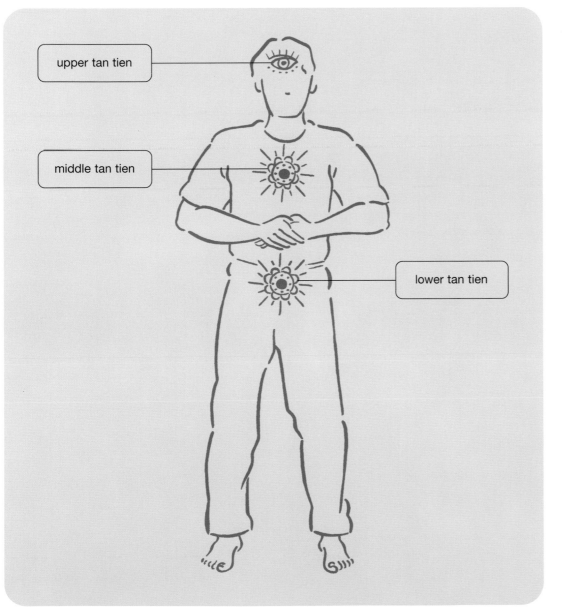

left: The Tan Tiens are the main energy centers of the body.

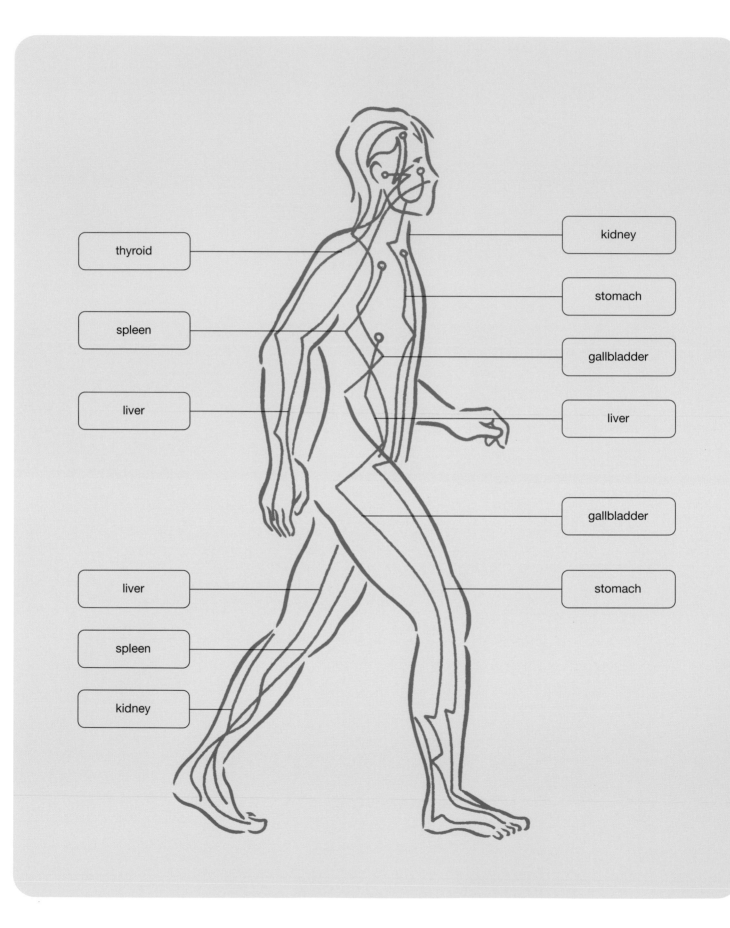

thyroid

spleen

liver

liver

spleen

kidney

kidney

stomach

gallbladder

liver

gallbladder

stomach

sexuality, and the essential emergency reserve of energy we have in times of crisis or illness. Regular practice of tai chi helps the energy to flow freely in, out, and around the Tan Tien (as well as elsewhere in the body); focusing the mind on the Tan Tien can further help chi to gather and eventually be absorbed and stored for use when needed. A famous tai chi master, Professor Cheng Man Ching, recommended focusing the mind at the Tan Tien all the time to make the best use of your time.

Along with this idea of storing and cultivating chi at the center of the body, the meridian (energy) lines of the body become less inhibited as blocks within them are dissolved, the chi beneath the muscles flows readily, and the chi of the internal organs is harmonized. At the very least, tai chi encourages the flow of life-giving energy and blood. Through the correct alignment of the energy centers, the energetic pathways are gradually strengthened and the flow of energy may increase, resulting in more vitality and radiant health. The energy system as a whole is enhanced and repaired and becomes more connected to the energy of the earth and heaven, much like a conduit for energy transmission.

tai chi and postural alignment

During the practice of tai chi we focus on aligning the body and holding postures. The body begins to correct itself of postural defects. Some of these effects can be seen over time as tension is released and areas of blockage are cleared. More entrenched postural misalignments may take many months—or even years—to correct. The essential points of tai chi encourage better posture and this benefits the musculoskeletal system. In my case, tai chi, massage, and Shiatsu (a traditional, hands-on Japanese healing therapy) have helped me improve my posture. Tai chi can really help with hunched shoulders and other postural problems and I have seen a lot of these problems lessened after several months of practice.

Good posture is essential for good health, as we rely on the functioning of the internal organs for our life. The spine is our essential support, holding the internal organs in place and carrying essential chi and electrical impulses from the brain to the rest of the body, and vice versa. The seated posture of tai chi helps improve breathing function, which improves the oxygenation of the blood. This posture also encourages diaphragmatic breathing, which, in turn, gently massages the internal organs. The posture itself also helps by maintaining the correct position of the organs, helping them work more effectively and without restriction.

left: The meridian lines trace the main channels of energy that course through the body.

Poor posture is indicative of a poor mental state. It inhibits energy flow and creates organ restriction; in turn, this creates blockage and eventually disease. Our bodies, in essence, also show our minds. A good posture is essential for psychological health.

In tai chi the basic posture is taken with the feet positioned a shoulder-width apart and pointing forward (anatomically correct and energetically neutral). The weight should go evenly through the feet and up through the knee and ankle joints. The knees should be soft and slightly bent (but not collapsed inward, as they should remain over the feet). The pelvis is tilted upward, the tailbone tucked in so the sacrum is flatter, and the lumbar region of the back should be straight. The body weight is sunk into the pelvic girdle and the hips. The belly should hang naturally and not be held in. The chest should be relaxed, so the breath can come into the whole of the lungs without restriction. The neck should be in line with the back and the chin tucked in slightly to help with this and to take the pressure off the occiput at the back of the neck. The tongue is placed on the roof of the mouth to connect the microcosmic orbit (see pages 60–61) and prevent the mouth from becoming too wet or too dry. As well as improving posture, this stance also aligns the body's energy and places you in balance between heaven and earth, facilitating a connection with the earth beneath your feet and the energy above your head.

Standing in any of the fixed postures is important for several reasons. First, the body and mind become familiar with the stances; second, the muscles are gradually strengthened; third, as the chi or energy begins to circulate, any blocked chi is released (this may produce spontaneous shaking); fourth, we develop mental as well as physical stamina. This traditional training method is used in most, if not all, styles and was as important, if not more important, than performing the sequences. In fact, this is really a foundation for form work and can also help to strengthen the connective tissues of the body.

Your postures should be erect yet relaxed,
    able to meet an attack from the eight directions.

Tai Chi Classics

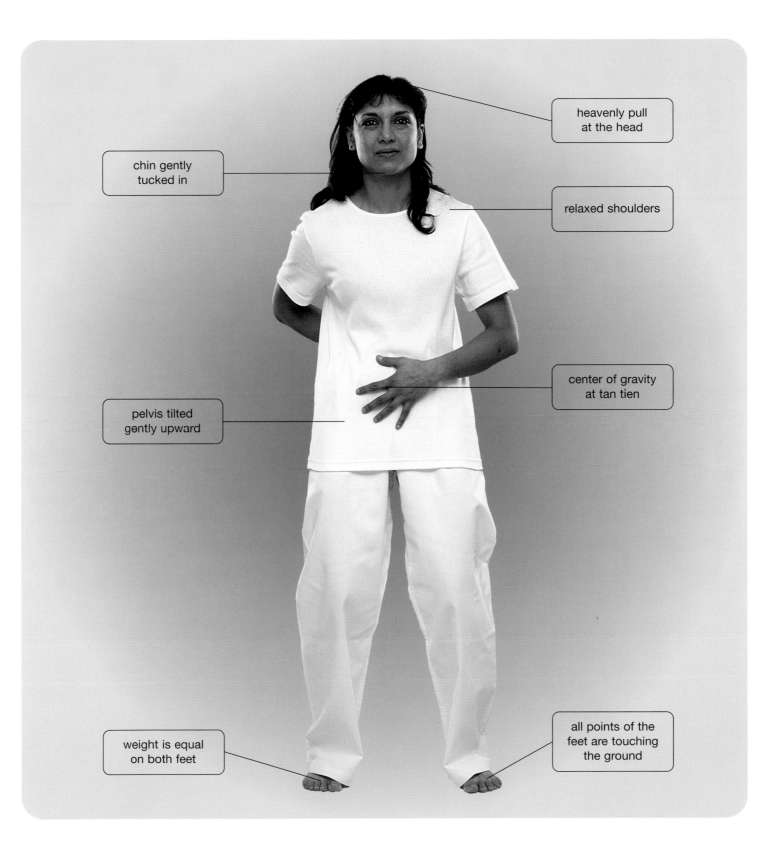

heavenly pull
at the head

chin gently
tucked in

relaxed shoulders

center of gravity
at tan tien

pelvis tilted
gently upward

weight is equal
on both feet

all points of the
feet are touching
the ground

above: This practitioner shows the perfect posture for tai chi: pelvis
lifted upward, tailbone tucked in, belly and chest relaxed.

rooting

By relaxing and sinking into the seated posture of tai chi, we lower our center of gravity and become more rooted. Being rooted, like a tree, is in a sense a by-product of applying the principles of tai chi within movement.

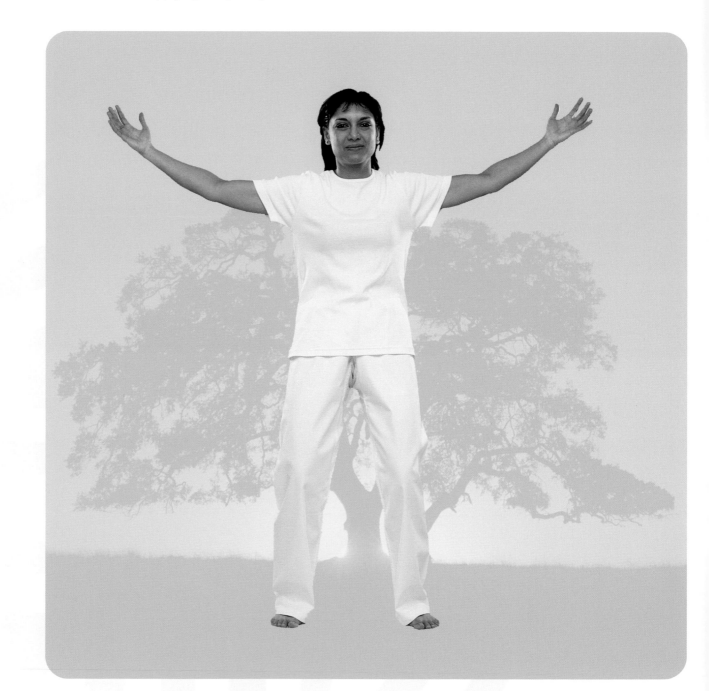

Gravity is the root of lightness.

Tao Te Ching, Verse 76

tai chi for a calmer mental state

When we focus inward, away from the distractions of daily life, and concentrate on beneficial objects such as our breathing, body, movement, or intent, then our mind naturally rebalances itself and we become more in tune with ourselves. The mind is freed from distractions and becomes aware of more subtle states of being, tuning into a more kinesthetic way of being. By practicing tai chi we become more present and focused on the here and now, the only moment that is real! One of the essential points of all tai chi styles is to practice with a calm mind. Tai chi cultivates this sense of calm within us while also strengthening our bodies.

Stress relief is one of the main reasons why people try tai chi. Because stress and repetitive strain injury are such big issues today, it is no surprise that businesses and organizations are looking to tai chi in an effort to negate the effects of both stress and stress-related illness. The learning process of tai chi has been used by companies as a way of building cooperation, team building, and bonding. How many relaxing things do we ever do with our colleagues?

Stress-related illness is the biggest single factor affecting absenteeism at work and it costs national economies billions every day. Fast living, enormous pressure, an uncertain future, security issues, crime, divorce, child rearing, mass consumerism, and ecological disaster all combine to make today's world probably the most stressful it has ever been. We seem to be living on the brink of one disaster or another, struggling to survive, working ever-increasing hours, and having less time to do more things.

For organizations that have a legal responsibility toward their employees, strategies to reduce the cost of absenteeism and damage caused by burnout, stress-related mental illness, and the enormous pressure of the business world are evolving all the time. People now frequently seek the help of counselors, Shiatsu masseurs, stress management consultants, and motivational gurus. These professionals are all lining up to impart knowledge, build team spirit, and reduce the effects of stress.

the importance of relaxation

Relaxation is as important as discipline and effort, in fact it takes discipline to be relaxed and it takes effort, too. In tai chi, the relaxation we are looking for is not "floppy" or collapsed, but rather a confident relaxation with inner strength and power drawn from within. Relaxation does not mean going to sleep or giving up; it means not trying too hard and just being you. Relaxation is at the heart of being confident and fearless. It is the by-product of success and craved by nearly everyone. Relaxation is an art; it is a component of discipline and a prerequisite for application that will help you attract what you want in life. Relaxation is a major component of tai chi and being happy.

The benefits of tai chi are in both the body and the mind. The object of our focus and concentration is our body, intent, and movement. This process of focusing inward helps us become free from distractions. In fact, it is impossible to worry about the past or future during tai chi practice. By leading the mind in this way, we become more present. The body is relaxed through the technique of posture and by the flowing movements. By correctly aligning the body it can relax more readily as the structures within the body become more supportive of each other. The muscular action of tai chi releases tension and stress-related aches and pains, thus further aiding the relaxation process. Relaxation is the key to "sinking" with the mind and energy—this is how we develop groundedness in practice and "rooting," the ability to be like a tree and to relax and sink into the seated posture. Often, relaxation and energy is the only emphasis in some tai chi schools, but this alone will not work and the movements will not be grounded. Tai chi postures are essentially very strong, but they must be flexible, too. Everything is about balance.

Chi flows more potently when we are relaxed. Tension and the use of force inhibits chi and makes us uptight and tired. When the muscles of the body are relaxed the chi can move and circulate freely, accumulating at the Tan Tien more readily. This ability to relax has a positive effect on our immune system, enabling it to remove toxins from the body and allowing blood to flow much more readily. By becoming more relaxed our breathing and oxygenation of blood improves, as does the body's ability to recover from hard physical or mental work and illness. Relaxed internal organs work better and digestion is more efficient and healthy when the nervous system is relaxed.

tai chi for meditation

In tai chi we develop the connection between mind and body in a meditative way. You can visualize the body as a sponge, the mind like water. By soaking the mind into the body our ability to perform tai chi gradually improves. The object of the meditation is the body and involves initially getting the basic moves right. At this stage we are developing kinesthetic awareness. Gradually, as our awareness and concentration grow,

left: Raise Hands is a good example of a stance that allows the body and mind to open and close in unity.

the movement becomes more clearly defined and more fluid so we can relax more.
When this happens we become more conscious and can work more effectively with
rooting and intent, the ability to focus mind and movement in a desired direction
or way, and eventually advance to opening and closing the body, mind, and energy.
Opening and closing is a martial technique where the whole body expands (opening) to
brush off an attack, or contracts (closing) around an arm to trap it. This process can be
seen in moves such as Ward Off and Raise Hands.

This mental training has many benefits, not least the ability to free the mind from
distraction and worry. This naturally makes the mind more peaceful. Tai chi is all in the
mind; at least it begins with the *hsin* (mind/heart or consciousness) and involves the
use of *yi* (intent) to guide the internal energy and the movement.

below: Visualization is an important part of tai chi meditation, and picturing calming scenes
immediately helps to slow down the heart rate.

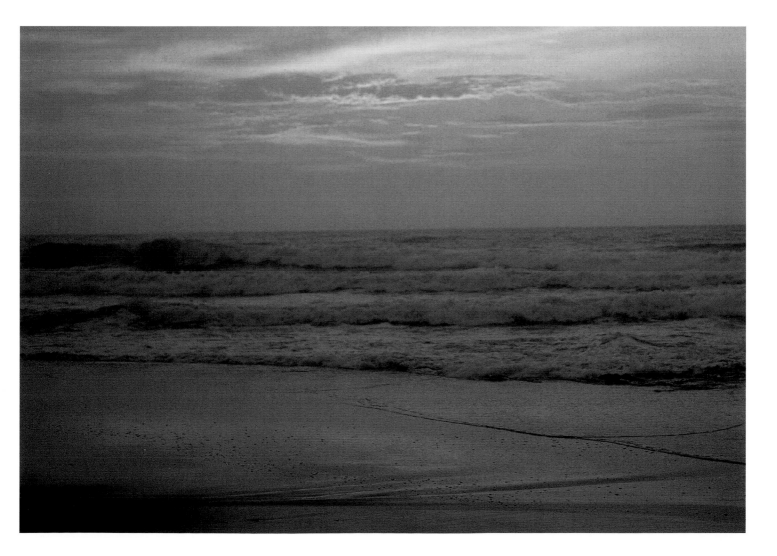

Mental benefits of tai chi:

• Development of concentration to learn the initial movements
• Mental relaxation necessary for refinement
• Development of mental awareness for "conscious movement"
• Deepening of mental aspects through understanding the eight energies of tai chi
• Mind and body harmony: Training the mind, the body follows, the energy follows, the spirit is raised
• Focus and intent
• Yi and li (Mind and internal force)
• Attitude, confidence, and awareness
• Practicing with a calm mind

The Yi, or mind, leads the Li, or internal force, and with awareness the whole process of mental training begins. Initially, the mind is trained just to learn the movements, and then the deeper aspects of cultivating, circulating, and directing energy can begin. Energy flow may well be noticeable at first but understanding how tai chi works as an internal art is a process that takes time and effort.

tai chi for the spirit

> The most important reason is that when you finally reach the place where you understand what life is about, you'll have the health to enjoy it.
>
> Master Cheng Man Ching

In Taoism there are numerous practices for attaining longevity, and ultimately immortality (transcending death through development of the conscious mind and energy/spiritual body). Tai chi masters are, and have always been, interested in "internal alchemy"—a way of influencing and cultivating vital, psychic, and spiritual energy for the purpose of prolonging life and improving one's state of mind. To a large degree they succeeded in improving their health, and may have even attained special powers to direct energy and heighten perception. In today's world, however, the alchemy we perhaps most crave is one that provides greater harmony, health, and well-being. This spiritual quest has become a well-worn path in the West since the 1960s. Many believe that Western religious institutions have failed to answer life's important questions and the movement toward seeking answers from Eastern philosophies and religions has grown, with tai chi being very much a part of this movement.

Spirit is commonly seen as either an expression of an altruistic idea (for example, human heroics or great achievement); as an expression of aliveness and vibrancy; or as an immortal part of us that survives death. It all depends on your point of view. Many people would see spirit in terms of a relationship with our creator, or as a form of discipline that unites body and mind to produce harmony and a sense of well-being (along with a transformation of attitude). Spiritually, tai chi offers us a way of calming the mind and becoming more aware of the subtle energies that flow within us, while also remaining grounded and relaxed. This paves the way within us to receive a more personal insight into our lives and a deeper awareness of nature, beauty, and mutual respect for others and ourselves.

Because tai chi is a form of meditation, it can help us deal with problems in a positive and constructive way. What you may believe on a spiritual level is entirely your own choice—and tai chi is not a religion.

The spirit of tai chi emerges after the mental, physical, and energetic elements become harmonized and unified. At this point the practitioner is working in harmony with himself and there is no longer any separation between the different aspects of practice. Whole-body movement led by consciousness becomes a reality and you begin to experience the flow without any need for a personal agenda. The mind is calm and the spirit is raised.

In tai chi, if you train the mind, the energy follows and so the spirit is raised. I would define "spirit" as the essential spark within each of us that is beyond the normal modes of time and space and is the mystical part of the tai chi journey. I remember once, when practicing tai chi after a class, my mind was very quiet, as it normally is when I practice, but this time I felt suddenly free from the agendas of my personality. Liberated and free within my body, I felt like a tai chi spiritual warrior in an almost enlightened state, without worry and totally present and in awe of life. I would describe this as a peak experience, but not a euphoric one. As a path to enlightenment, tai chi in itself is, I believe, not enough, but there is no doubt in my mind that as an aid to inner peace and harmony it is a huge gift to mankind.

tai chi as a martial art

> ## Can you make your body as soft and supple as that of a child?
>
> Lao Tzu

As a fighting art, tai chi has nothing to do with force and aggression. It has everything to do with a relaxed mind and body—and the deeply philosophical approach of overcoming aggression with calmness. It is a way of using your skills, rather than your physical strength, to resolve conflict. As a system of close-quarter natural combat, it calls for a relaxed body and mental state. From this calmness comes great speed and effective deflection. Rather than use brute force to overcome an attacker, the aggressor's own force is turned back on them to subdue them with minimum effort.

The person lunging forcefully toward you will have lost their center of gravity—and therefore their advantage. It is also likely that they will be focusing all their strength in one very specific part of their body—a hand or a foot—and once that force has been expended in a blow, they are temporarily without strength. And that is when the tai chi practitioner reacts. Pushing, pulling, locking, or throwing are all designed to neutralize an attack without inflicting too serious an injury.

Practicing the slow forms teaches you the technique of relaxing, and this will eventually enable you to execute the forms at speed while your inner being remains totally calm.

Ultimately, martial art training is about much more than self defense. It is about self development, learning to recognize and counter our weaknesses, developing a calm mind, and treating others with dignity and compassion.

All styles of tai chi can be used for effective self defense. The main difference between tai chi self defense and, for example, kung fu or karate, is that it takes longer to see and feel how it can be truly effective. For this and other reasons, such as personal inclination, many tai chi instructors do not understand the martial side of tai chi, or even wish to. However, it should be remembered that tai chi without martial skill (either for fighting or as a strategy for interaction) is not really tai chi. In essence, the true martial power of tai chi takes many years to master but the simple techniques are fairly easy to grasp.

The characteristics of tai chi as a martial art:

• Using softness to overcome hardness

• Not retaliating (or fighting force with force)

• Yielding like a sapling

• Listening (aurally, visually, via body language, and sensing a mental/physical attack before it happens) to anticipate an attack

• Using the Eight Energies (see pages 42–45) of tai chi and Fa Jin (the technique of releasing power through a synergy of sinking, opening, technique, and mental intent)

tai chi moves for self-defense

• **Parting the Wild Horse's Mane:** Here, yielding and turning the waist is used as the attack comes in. The fist is redirected away from the body with the right hand. The left arm comes up and inside the attacker's right arm and the attacker is drawn in close. Meanwhile, the shoulder is used in conjunction with a grip. A step onto the right leg of the attacker is used and the attacker is pulled off balance. As the waist turns, the attacker is thrown to the left and defeated.

• **White Crane:** A double deflection and kick are used in response to two punches. The attacking energy is split and a kick is used to attack.

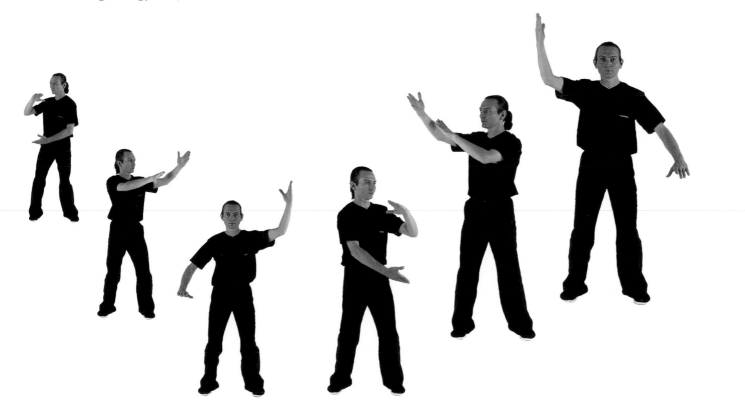

above: White Crane is a classic tai chi form for self-defense.

a summary of the benefits of tai chi

more energy

The fluid movements of tai chi, along with the energetic and physical alignments, are designed to increase energy flow and release energy blocks and tension, giving you more vitality and energetic balance. Physically, you become fitter and stronger; gradually and gently, you become more energized. The breathing aspect leads to increased lung elasticity and improved oxygenation of the blood, increasing energy to the brain and muscles. Visualization techniques can help relax and energize the body.

improved ability to concentrate

The subtle mental training within tai chi develops mental focus. Practicing leads to an improved ability to concentrate. The improved breathing leads to improved oxygenation of the blood and improved brain function.

less stress

A more relaxed you is a less stressed you. The combination of improved relaxation and physical health greatly influences emotional equanimity and therefore lessens adverse reaction to stress. When the mind is free from worry there is no need to fear anything. A positive attitude equals raised spirits, which equals less worry.

calmness

Mind-body harmony + meditative qualities of tai chi = calm.

better health

Many physical problems manifest themselves when there is poor circulation, a run-down immune system, and negative mental thinking. By improving the blood circulation, stimulating the body's natural defenses, and imbuing the mind with positive qualities, tai chi is the ideal tonic and preventative measure against poor health.

happiness

The ultimate human goal is to be happy, or at least to move toward that goal. When we are not happy we know about it because we suffer. Therefore, cultivating the conditions for happiness—and enjoyment—to grow are essential for your personal development and fulfillment. Such needs should not be left unfulfilled. Tai chi practice is one way to help yourself and those around you lead a happier life.

mental clarity

Practicing concentration and developing focus in a relaxed way will undoubtedly lead to an improved state of mind. The Taoist way of the "middle path" is in part about finding mental equanimity and becoming clearer and more balanced. Tai chi practice leads to clearer thinking and fewer disorganized thoughts.

less back pain

Back pain is one of the scourges of modern times. It costs us millions, causes us a lot of pain, and can become a recurring nightmare for millions of people. Overwork, poor posture, accidents, and emotional blockage are some of the causes. Tai chi strengthens the core stability muscles in the mid- to lower back, tones the muscles in the upper back, and improves posture, body (kinesthetic) awareness, and spatial awareness, thus lessening the risk of back problems and improving rate and chance of recovery.

more time and time for self

More quality time is always being sought. A more relaxed and confident you will make you worry less about time, enjoy the time you do have, and will allow you to make the right decisions at the right time—and by default creating more quality time for yourself. Tai chi also gives you time to focus on yourself in a positive way, recharging your batteries, and helping yourself relax.

below: Tai chi encourages you to be rooted like a tree, and believes that by developing inner strength and power you can find happiness and relaxation.

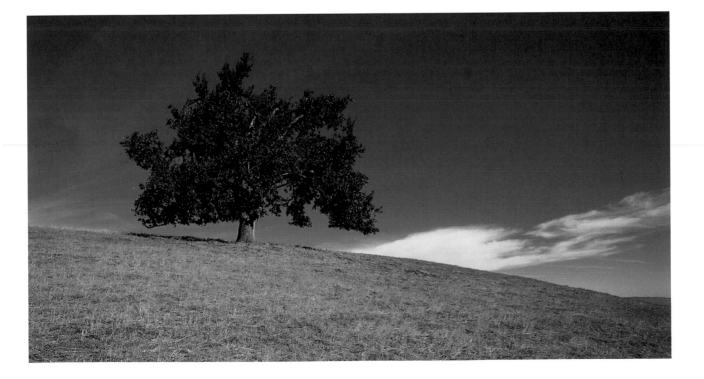

the eight energies

One of the unique features of tai chi is the Eight Energies. These are, in essence, eight techniques of intent, energetic expression, and movement that produce a particular effect in form and Push Hands practice. They are all related and can flow and change into one another. These are traditionally the techniques used with energy in a martial context but also form a part of advanced form, Push Hands, and martial arts practice.

The Eight Energies relate to the essential "why?" of a movement and can give real meaning to your practice. With practice and study you will be able to recognize each of the eight phases within your own movements.

peng (ward off)

Peng is the energetic platform that all the other energies are based on. Peng is often described as an upward-expanding energy and can be compared to the pressure in a tire wall or inflatable boat. In the movement, Ward Off is shown as it appears in the form. This quality helps you keep your shape and avoid collapsing. As a principle, though, Peng should be present in all your tai chi practice.

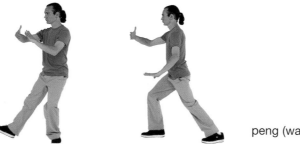

peng (ward off)

lu (roll back)

This technique uses qualities of absorption and redirection to deal with an incoming force. When yielding and dispersing an attack, while parrying that force, Lu is used as a way of negating an attack.

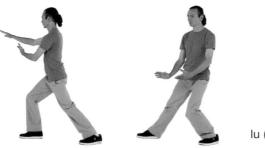

lu (roll back)

ji (press)

A direct force when issued in a straight line and using relaxed internal power. An outwardly expressed force, Ji is a classic example of using Fa Jin in an overt way, almost like an arrow leaving a bow.

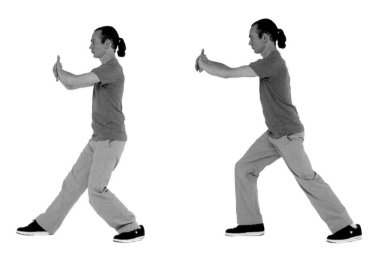

ji (press)

an (push)

When we yield and push down on an incoming attack to break down its root, this is known as *An*. We can then choose to push the attacker away as they will be easily uprooted. Expert timing is needed for this push before the attacker has regained their root and balance.

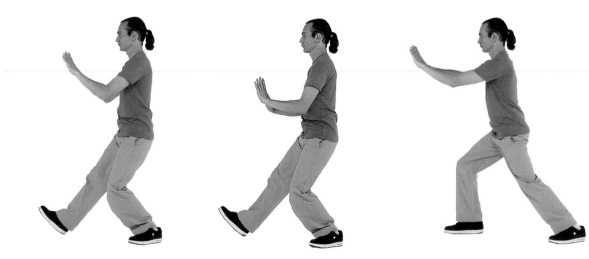

an (push)

tsai (pull down)

To turn an opponent and direct them downward is known as *Tsai*. By maintaining your shape and turning like a sphere on its central axis, it is possible to deflect a lot of energy while using little of your own. Tsai employs this technique to great effect. It can be seen in the transition into White Crane Spreads Its Wings.

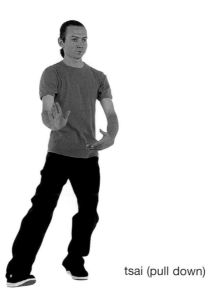

tsai (pull down)

lieh (split)

Lieh can be used explosively to split an incoming force. Two energies are moved simultaneously in opposite directions by pulling, redirecting, or moving in opposite directions. This can be seen in the transition into Single Whip, Repulse the Monkey, and Fan Penetrates the Back.

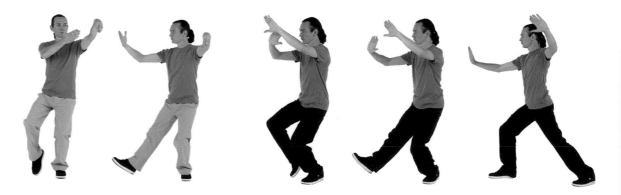

lieh (split)—single whip   lieh (split)—fan penetrates the back

lieh (split)—repulse the monkey

kao (shoulder strike)

In the Chen style of tai chi the obvious spiraling movements that flow through the shoulders, with the intention of directing energy from there, is known as *Kao*. This technique is also shown in the other styles, but not so overtly. In the transition from Raise Hands to White Crane Spreads Its Wings, Kao is used to deflect an attacker.

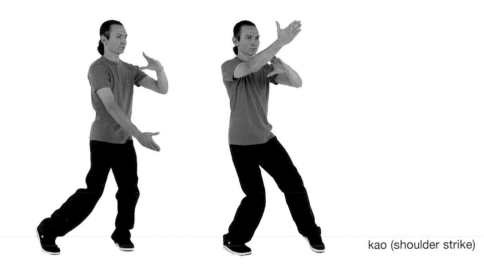

kao (shoulder strike)

jou (elbow strike)

This is very similar to Kao, except the elbow is used. The energized movements make use of the whole body, including the hips and other joints. The waist is seen as the director of this movement and the whole process can be used either therapeutically for health or for defensive and attacking movements. With Jou, the intended movement is focused through the elbow to either strike outward or to evade a grip.

tai chi martial principles for interpersonal skills

Good employers serve their workers.

Tao Te Ching, Verse 68, "Good Warriors"

As a beneficial and rebalancing activity, tai chi has a lot to offer business organizations that are committed to reducing stress-related illnesses and musculoskeletal disorders. The refreshing sensation of tai chi provides more energy and a more effective approach to problem-solving. Recent studies have shown that tai chi has a marked effect on brain waves. Normally, the brain functions on an alpha frequency (an active state) but changes to a beta (receptive/passive) state when we are relaxed.

While in the beta state, the brain is more responsive to new information and retention of information is also improved. Tai chi practice has been proven to change brain waves from alpha to beta, making it useful as a way of supporting learning.

not fighting force with force

One of the fundamental principles of martial tai chi is not to fight force with force, but to use flexibility, yielding, and redirecting to overcome an attack. To do this effectively you need to remain centered, even under duress. Taking this idea and using it as a life skill can enhance your interpersonal relationships as well as your effectiveness in dealing with stressful situations. For example, when handling a difficult customer, colleague, or business partner, it is best not to add to the negativity of the situation by just trying to win the argument. In situations of conflict, the other person's story is as relevant as your own (even if you may not think so at the time), so it serves you to know what they have to say.

remaining centered

By remaining centered (see Focusing at the Tan Tien, pages 27–29) we can avoid extremes of anger and overactivity. We naturally become more patient and in the present. This may also help us in situations where we tend to become nervous. Because the mind's tendency is to go from one thing to another, sometimes in an out-of-control way, any technique that gives us more mental control is especially effective.

yielding and listening

The person you are dealing with has valuable information. By listening to what he is saying, you equip yourself to deal effectively with the problem. By yielding (not fighting but remaining strong, like a sapling, for example) you give him the space to express what he wants. Finding out where your client is coming from is facilitated through the process of listening and holding your ground, but being flexible means that you can be the other winner in the situation by making yourself heard, too.

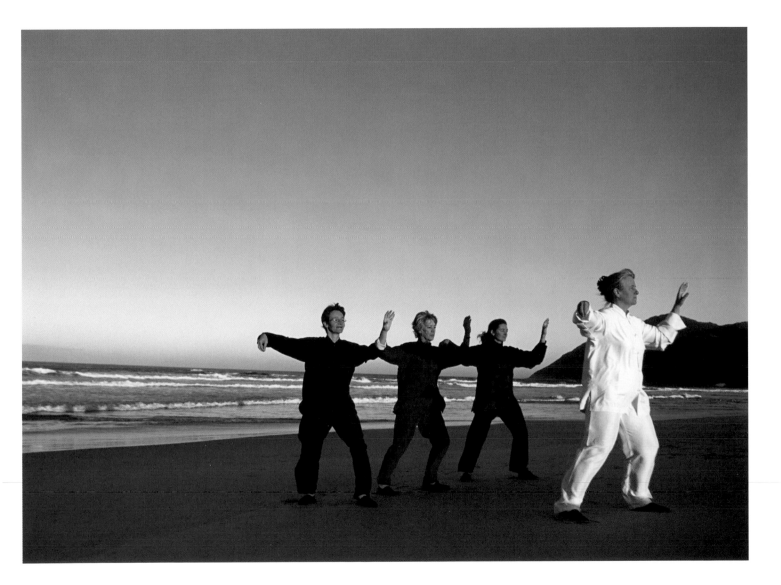

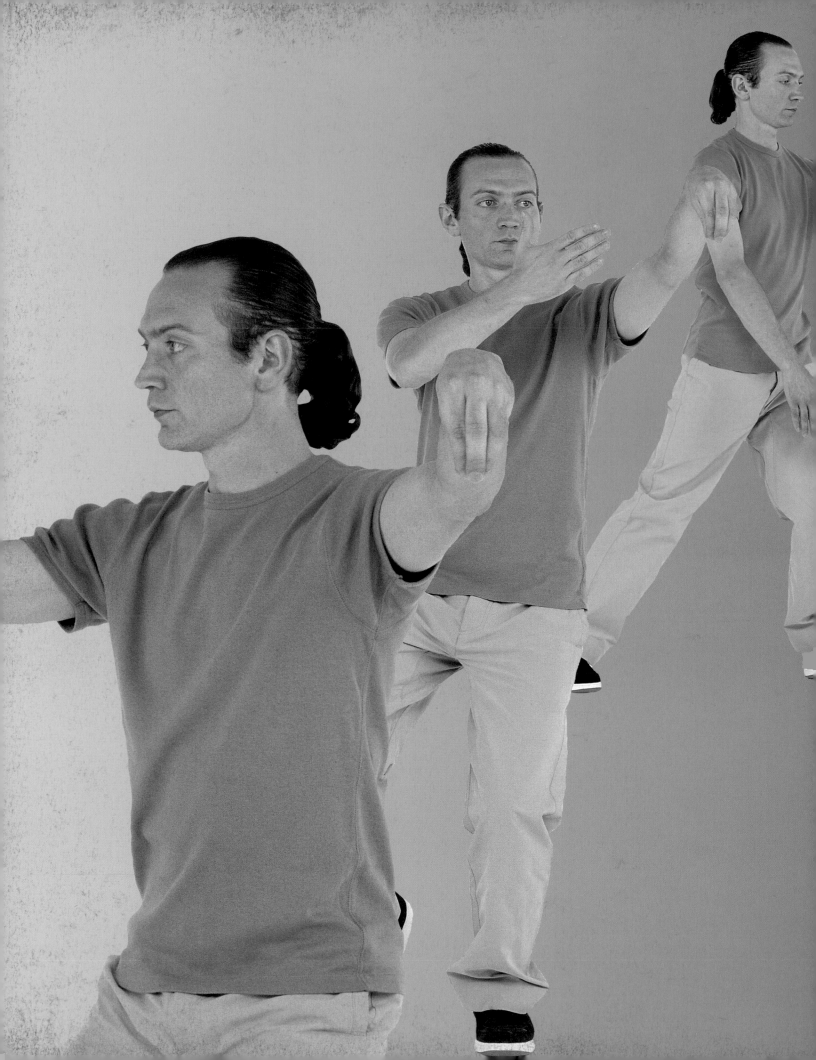

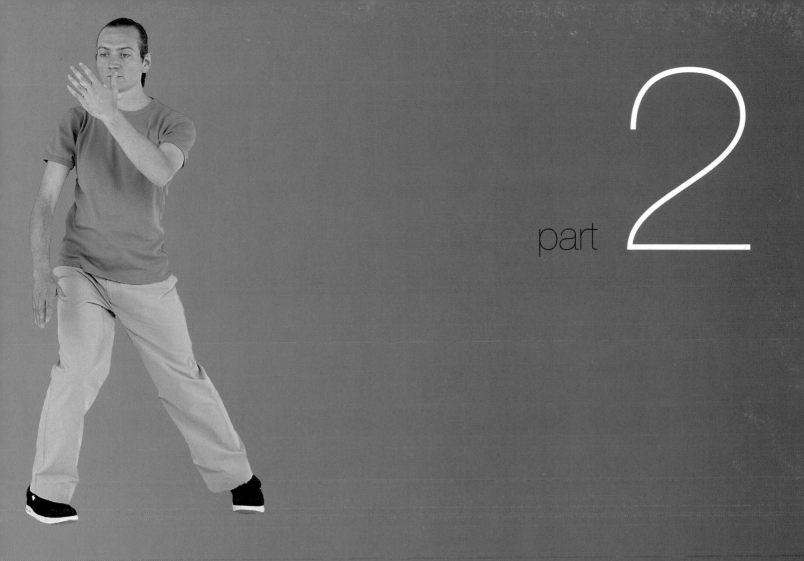

tai chi in practice

A way can be a guide, but not a fixed path;
names can be given but not permanent labels.

Tao Te Ching, Verse 1, "A Way Can Be a Guide"

essential guidance for
tai chi practice

the ten-point practice

All the movements in tai chi are done at a slow pace. This is to assist concentration and develop kinesthetic awareness. The muscles are encouraged to relax so that the movements are free from tension and awkwardness. The turning of the body is done on the central axis and is directed with the waist. When turning, avoid twisting your body and turn your hips and shoulders together. The hands should be relaxed and open, with the fingers not held closely together. This will encourage the energy to flow and the acupuncture points, such as the Loa Gong, to open. Above all, take your time and enjoy your practice.

Yang Cheng Fu (1883–1936), a tai chi master, originally compiled the following ten points of guidance for tai chi practice. They are concise and easy-to-follow, making them ideal as a framework for initial practice. This list is based on several translations, as well as my own experience with them. You can choose to use them as a basis for your practice once you have learned the basic moves. Tai chi is the synergy of all these points, so each part is related to another.

the energy at the top of the head should be light

The position of the head is very important and can affect the quality of your movement. When the head is relaxed and in line with the neck and back, the subtle energies within the body can circulate freely. The chin is tucked in very slightly to take pressure off the occiput, located at the back of the head, at the top of the neck. As the head is about as heavy as bowling ball, this helps to facilitate the feeling of lightness at the top of the head. This lightness can be helped by visualizing a golden thread gently pulling you upward from the top of your head. Some teachers also describe this as gently pushing upward from inside, or as growing. As you do this, you relax the waist and tuck the tailbone in as you tilt the pelvis upward. The overall effect of this is a confident, relaxed posture that feels connected and grounded.

sink the chest and raise the back

Sinking means to relax downward through the body by consciously softening the muscles so the energy can move freely and gather at the Tan Tien, located just below the navel. The raising of the back is the upward movement through the spine that occurs as the posture and the waist sink. The base of the spine is pulled downward and the crown of the head rises, so the whole back is lengthened in two directions. This is not possible without relaxing and sinking (but not collapsing) the chest.

relax the waist

When the pelvis is tilted and you sink into the posture as if sitting, it is necessary to relax the waist and sink into the pelvic girdle. This is how the posture is stacked up and it will create a stable foundation for movement. The waist directs the movements of the arms while we turn on the central axis of the body. The motion of the whole movements in tai chi is said to be rooted in the feet, transmitted through the legs, directed by the waist, and manifested in the fingers. The waist therefore is seen as the governor of the movement and the fulcrum is at the Tan Tien. Everything moves together as a whole, so the waist must be relaxed in order to keep the movements fluid and changing.

distinguish between substantial and insubstantial

Tai chi stances are either solid or empty, with one leg more heavily planted into the ground than the other. When we take a step out, the placement of the foot on the ground is like a cat: No weight or force comes forward until the foot is placed. This helps you to be more in control of the movements. It also promotes ease of movement and stability. If this is not the case, the movements become clumsy. By practicing in this way we can improve the relaxed strength of the legs and become more conscious of our movements. Distinguishing between full and empty is also essential for understanding how tai chi works in relation to the philosophical basis as set down in *The Tai Chi Classics*, the collected writings of tai chi masters thought to date from the time of the Chan Sang Feng.

sinking the shoulders and the elbows

By sinking the shoulders our energy can circulate freely and our chi will not rise, making us top-heavy. The waist and Tan Tien are the central areas to where the chi must sink. If the elbows are not kept down and relaxed, the shoulders will rise and we will become tense. Relaxing the shoulders and elbows will add to the ease of movement.

using the mind instead of force

Tai chi movements are seemingly soft and fluid, with the use of tense, muscular force avoided. The initial training starts in the mind. The movements are done slowly so that we can guide them with the conscious mind and our intent. Without intent the movements become sloppy; with excessive effort and concentration we become tense. Finding a balance between mind, intent, and movement will lead us toward a true harmony of mind, body, and spirit, and we can become capable of progression. Several years of practice gives you the relaxed body of a master, but this is only the outside; inside, the body becomes strong and vibrant. Initially, it is necessary to relax as much as possible, using the mind to aid this process through awareness. One image that may be useful is to see the mind as water and the body as a sponge (see pages 34–35). In this way the movement becomes more conscious and controlled.

coordination of the upper and lower body

The motion begins in the feet, is propelled with the legs, directed by the waist, and is seen in the fingers—thus showing that the whole body is connected and set off like a chain reaction. Each part affects the other and the arms and legs are connected as if by ropes and pulleys. Any change in one part of the body creates changes throughout the system. When this happens, the body becomes truly responsive and the movement is unhindered. It is this smoothness and flow that makes tai chi unique.

unify the internal with the external

In the external form (sequence of movements) the movements are said to be full and empty, open and closed. This basic pattern of change is at the heart of tai chi. These four elements (full, empty, open, and closed) can be seen as outer manifestations of what the mind is doing and what the intent is directing. When the mind is directed in a particular way, the energy follows and we have a union of mind, body, and energy. When everything is in proper harmony the spiritual aspect becomes apparent.

continuous movement

The movements should be continuous and flowing, like a river. There is no break in this continuity and no exhaustion of our energy. This flow may have punctuation points at the end of the movement but there is no pause in the flow. The constant flow of tai chi imbues a sense of unity with one's self and the outer world as it dissolves the energy blockages within the meridians and gives a sense of joy.

stillness in movement

The slower we practice tai chi, the quieter our mind becomes. When the mind is still and in a state of equanimity the chi can sink toward the Tan Tien. This soothes both the body and mind. The "stillness" refers mainly to the mind, as in meditation. Tai chi is meditation within movement.

preparing for tai chi

where should I practice?

You can practice tai chi virtually anywhere within reason, as long as you have a flat area that is free from clutter. The two forms in this book can be done in an area the size of an average living room or outside on the lawn. It is best to avoid practicing outside in strong wind or if it is very damp, but in good weather, practice is enhanced by being outside, surrounded by the elements and fresh air. Since good air is so vital for health, it is best to practice in a well-ventilated room. Some people also prefer to avoid practicing under fluorescent lighting or near strong electromagnetic radiation (such as near power and telephone lines). Quiet is also a big factor, especially at first when you are developing your ability to concentrate and calm your mind. The more peaceful and unpolluted, the better.

do I need special clothes?

In a nutshell, no. As long as your clothes allow freedom of movement and are not restrictive in any way, you can wear just about anything. There are no special clothes you need to buy. As far as footwear is concerned, flat-soled shoes are best, and bare feet or socks are fine, too. Avoid heavy shoes with thick soles or heels of any kind, as these will adversely affect your posture.

what do I need to practice?

All you need is yourself and a book, video, or the guidance of a decent teacher. There is no equipment to buy, and no mats are needed. You may wish to buy some relaxing music to practice with, and there are some pleasant CDs available written specifically for tai chi practice.

when should I practice?

Whenever you have the time. It is best to create some time in your day when you will not be interrupted by other people or the phone ringing. Try to build tai chi practice into your daily schedule. Mornings and evenings are often the best times.

how often?

This is entirely up to you. Ideally, a practice session in the morning and evening is a good start. About forty minutes a day is fine, but even five or ten minutes is beneficial. The more you practice, the more you will benefit. Practicing when you first wake up in the morning will really set you up for a positive day. During lunch breaks (before eating) is a great time, and practicing before bed will ensure you have a good night's sleep.

warming up

These simple exercises are designed to warm up the muscle groups and loosen the main joints of the body. Warm-up exercises are also useful for freeing up tension and the blocked energy associated with it.

The movements in this chapter are an ideal introduction to the art of tai chi and can be practiced by themselves. They will effectively stretch and warm up many of the muscle groups, open up the energetic pathways of the body, and work on some of the key accupressure points, enhancing health and well-being.

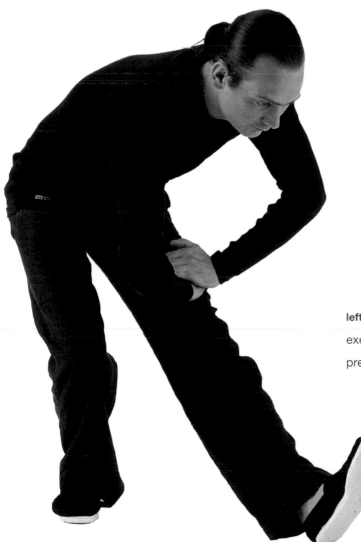

left: The Leg Stretch is one of the fundamental warm-up exercises, stretching and warming the leg muscles in preparation for tai chi.

warm-up exercises

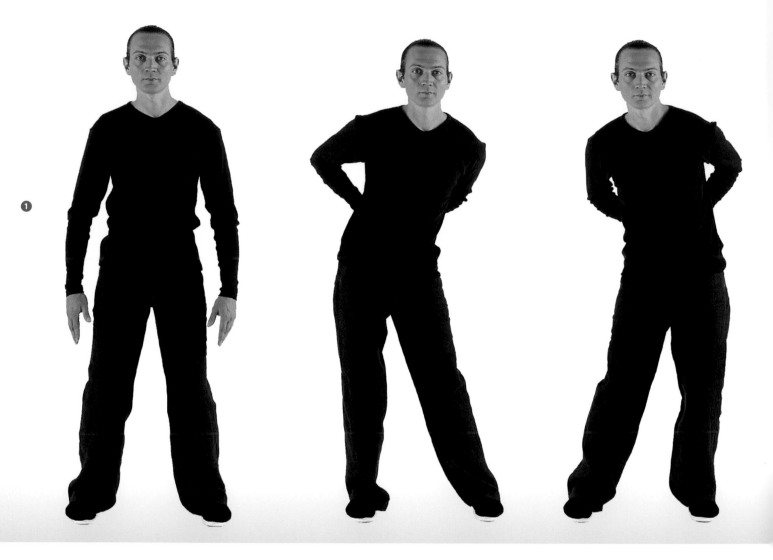

1 hip rolling

This exercise is designed to loosen up the hips and warm up the lower back. Start with your feet facing forward, shoulder-width apart, with the knees slightly bent.

Place your palms on the small of your back and guide your hips around in a circular movement at a slow, relaxed pace. Repeat this in the opposite direction.

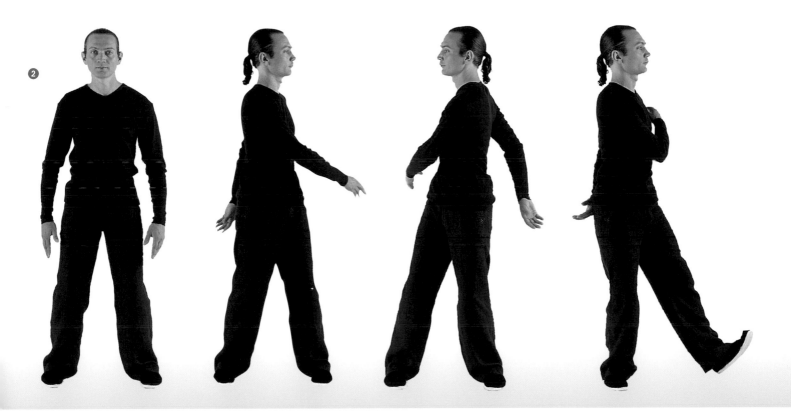

❷ turning from the waist

This exercise is great for warming up the center of the body, encouraging your arms to relax, and for familiarizing yourself with directing movement from your waist, one of the essential points of tai chi. It is also good for your back, and can encourage the flow of energy in the bladder meridian, one of the main outer energy channels of the body.

Beginning with your feet shoulder-width apart and facing forward, relax your knees so your stance is strong but relaxed.

Keep your back upright and your head level.

Turning on your central axis, relax your arms so they swing as you turn. Relax and turn from your waist. Repeat this movement a few times.

Begin to shift your weight into your right leg as your turn to the left, and your left leg as your turn to the right. Extend the movement further by turning your foot on the heel.

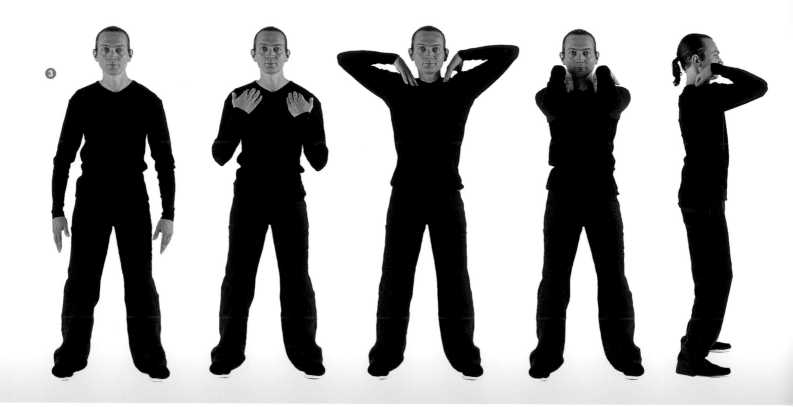

❸ shoulder circles

These are ideal for releasing tension and stress from the shoulders, as they warm up the joints and muscles. This is also very good for the lungs when the movement is reversed.

Place your fingers on your collarbone and bring your elbows down, back slightly, and then up, inward, and down, so you make a circular movement with your elbows.

Repeat this several times. You can coordinate this with your breath: Breathe in with the upward movement, and down with the downward movement. Repeat in the opposite direction.

❹ wrist and ankle rotations

These rotations are great for releasing blocks from these joints. It can also help to prevent pain caused by typing.

Interlock your fingers and move upward from your wrist joint and then outward in a circular fashion.

At the same time, circle one of your ankles. Repeat using the other ankle.

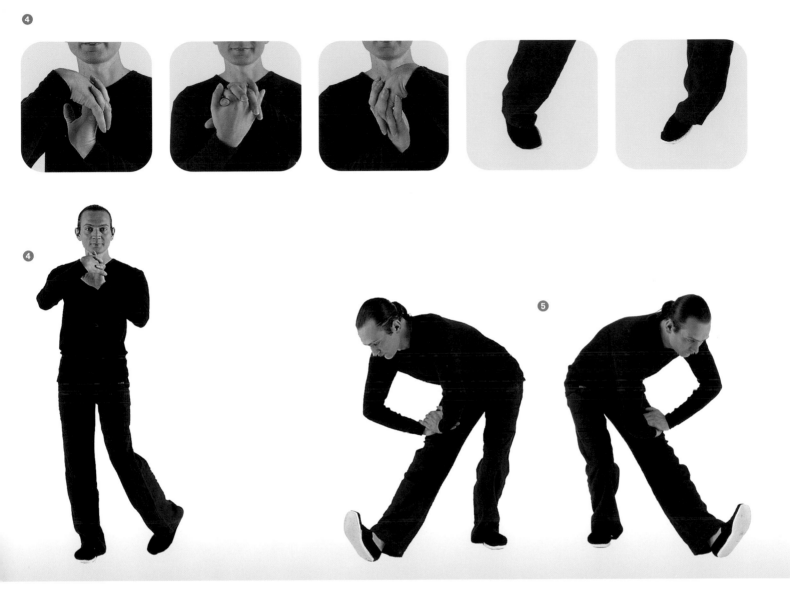

❺ leg stretches

These stretches will warm up the calf and other leg muscles while working on the bladder meridian, which runs down the back of the leg. These will also increase flexibility.

Start with your feet together and turn your left foot out about forty-five degrees. Take a natural step out and place your heel on the ground. Bring your toes back toward you.

Place your palms on your thigh, as shown, and bend from your waist, gently pressing into your thigh with your hands. You should feel a good stretch on the back of the leg. Release the stretch slowly and carefully.

Repeat for the other leg, then repeat the whole process, this time extending and deepening the stretch.

breathing exercises **with simple chi kung**

Chi Kung literally means "energy work" and it is a method of improving relaxation and the flow of internal energy. There are hundreds of Chi Kung exercises, which range from the elaborate and esoteric to the simple and basic. These two exercises are simple, yet highly effective for increasing well-being and a sense of centeredness. They serve as an excellent preparation for tai chi and can be done at any time of the day (except for the hour immediately after eating).

holding the ball chi kung

Stand with your feet shoulder-width apart and facing forward. "Sit" into your posture, tilting the pelvis upward and tucking in your tailbone. "Sink" and relax into your hips and relax your chest and shoulders. Tuck your chin in slightly to take the pressure off the occiput. Place your tongue on the roof of your mouth so you connect the internal energy channel (microcosmic orbit). Breathe in and out through your nose. Pay attention to the sensations in your body. Breathe naturally with your diaphragm. You may notice your abdomen rise and fall with your breathing.

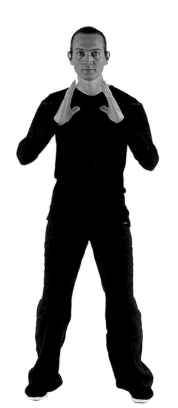

❷ Focus your attention on the sensations in your hands, and as you breathe in, allow the imaginary ball to expand to shoulder width. As you breathe in, try to feel your whole body gently expand. Imagine positive energy and vitality filling your body. As you breathe out, relax and let go of any negative thoughts.

❶ Let your hands rise up to about shoulder height and bring them in toward your chest, as if holding a ball.

the microcosmic orbit: an internal energy channel The microcosmic orbit is a channel of energy that runs down the front and up the back of the central axis (the spine, neck, and skull) of the body via energetic gateways, including the Tan Tien, situated just below the navel, and the Ming Men, located between the second and third lumbar vertebrae. This channel is gently strengthened by the posture of tai chi, leading to greater well-being and the flow of life-giving energy. There are specific meditations for developing the flow of energy in this channel, which are more suitable for advanced practitioners, rather than for beginners. The meditations in this book, however, are suitable for beginners.

holding the tan tien

Stand with your palms placed over your Tan Tien (located just below your navel). Relax and pay attention to the sensations within your body beneath your hands. Try to maintain this focus for about three or four minutes. When you have finished, slowly open your eyes and bring your attention back into the present moment.

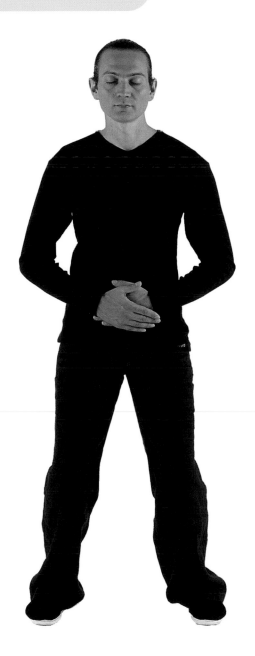

simple upper-body
tai chi movements

These eight movements are designed as an introduction to practice and as a primer for form work. Each exercise will familiarize you with the basics needed for learning a complete form and will help you develop a working awareness of some of the principles of tai chi practice. By themselves, they are very beneficial—particularly if you are limited in terms of space or do not have time to learn a complete form yet. As a step in your process of learning, they are an invaluable set of accessible and relaxing movements.

1. open tai chi

The general feeling here is like sitting down on a stool and placing your palms on a table in front of you. The stance should feel rooted, connected, and grounded, almost as if you are growing roots into the ground while growing upward through the crown of your head. The finished posture could be described as being between heaven and earth.

This movement is very calming and will strengthen the lower back muscles, improve postural awareness, and enhance the circulation of your blood and chi. (To practice this movement as a Chi Kung exercise, breathe in with the upward movement and out with the downward movement.)

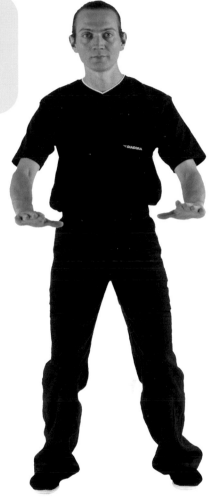

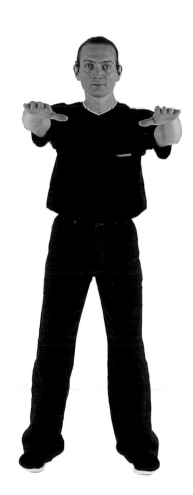

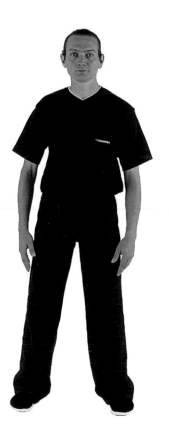

❶ Start with your feet shoulder-width apart and facing forward, with your arms relaxed by your sides.

❷ Raise your hands to shoulder height (as if you are underwater and your arms are floating to the surface of the water), your fingers and arms naturally extended. Your palms should come to shoulder height and face the floor.

❸ Bend your elbows and press down through the air with your palms. Relax your shoulders and sit into your stance. Bend the knees, keep your back raised (as if being pulled upward from the top of your head) and straight. Be aware of the sensations in your body. Repeat by raising the palms and straightening the legs.

2. parting the wild horse's mane

The martial technique of this movement is a throw (see page 166). In essence, the first part (Holding the Ball) is closed; the second part (Parting the Wild Horse's Mane) is open. This movement involves turning the body on its central axis, directing movement with the waist, and turning the hips and shoulders together. You should avoid twisting your body. Turn evenly and gently, but with intent. Parting the Wild Horse's Mane is very good for the digestive system, as the movement gently massages the internal organs. All the points of posture previously described apply to this and all subsequent movements.

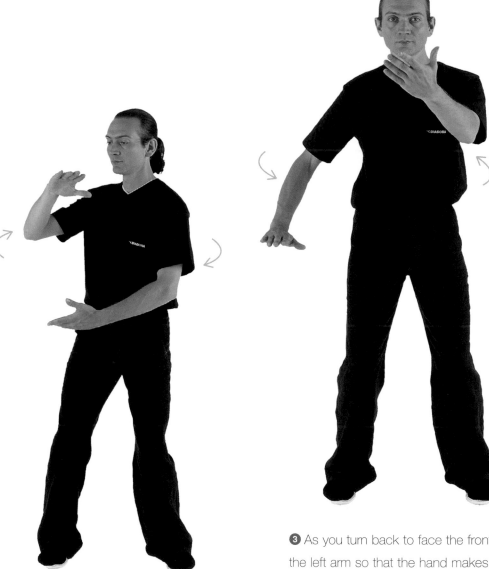

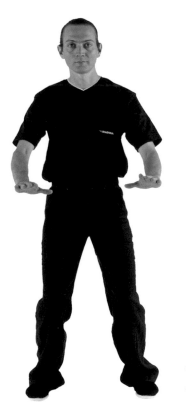

❶ Begin as if you have finished the first movement.

❷ Turn to your right, raising your right palm to form the top of a large, imaginary ball. Turn the left palm upward and bring it directly beneath the right palm.

❸ As you turn back to face the front, raise the left arm so that the hand makes an arc. Stroke your right palm downward, to hip height. The left palm is now straight in front of you, facing in, but slightly outward.

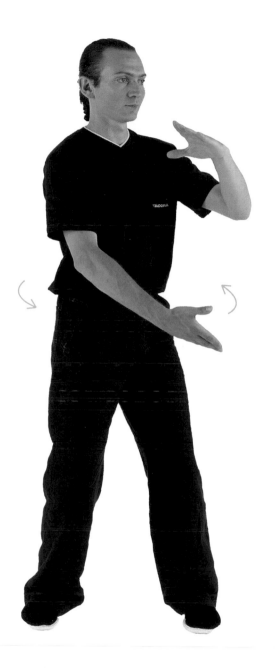

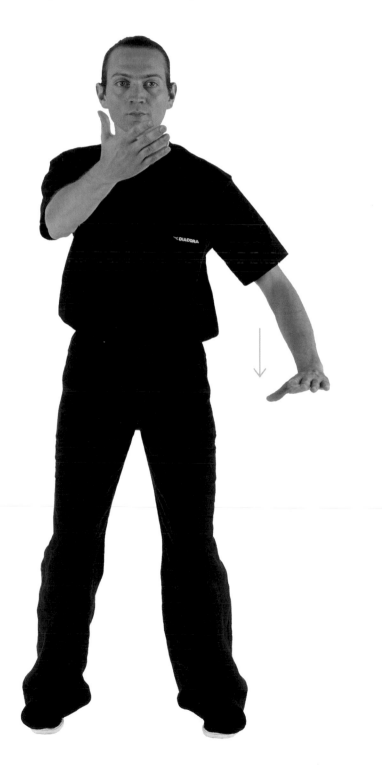

5 Stroke downward toward the side of the body with the left hand. From here, simply turn to the right again, hold the ball, and then turn back to the front, raising the left hand and stroking downward with the right hand as before. Repeat in sequence until your movements begin to flow. Remember to turn the body simultaneously with the movements of your hands and arms.

4 From here, turn to the left, turning the left palm so that it forms the top of the ball, and bringing the right palm around so that it is underneath. As you turn to the front, raise your right palm upward in an arc, with the palm facing in.

3. white crane

This movement is very open, expansive, and expressive. You can use your imagination. Imagine you are a bird such as a crane, stork, or heron, opening your wings to cool and air your feathers or to protect yourself from attack. The crane, when seen fighting with a snake, was one of the original inspirations for tai chi.

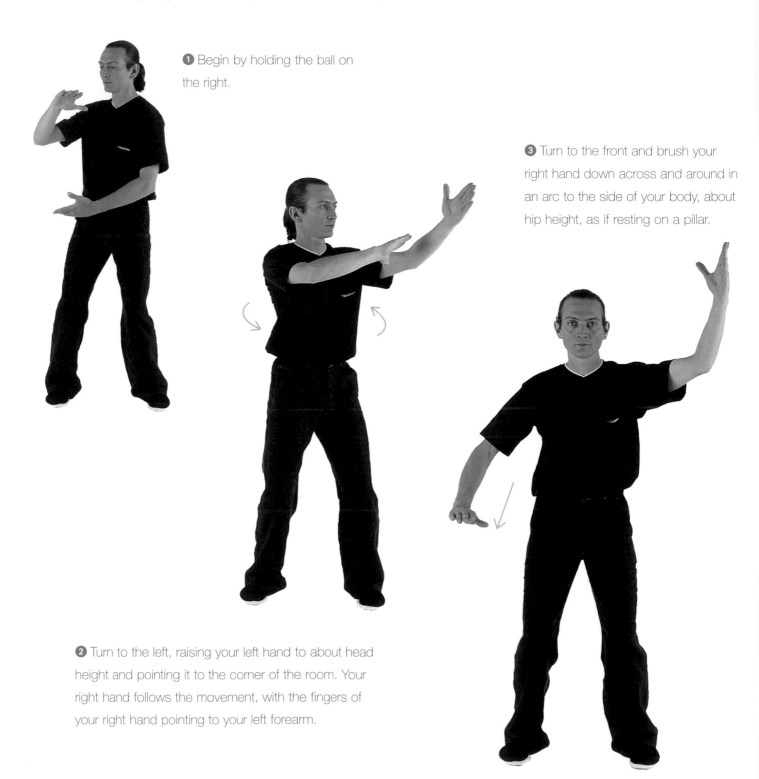

❶ Begin by holding the ball on the right.

❸ Turn to the front and brush your right hand down across and around in an arc to the side of your body, about hip height, as if resting on a pillar.

❷ Turn to the left, raising your left hand to about head height and pointing it to the corner of the room. Your right hand follows the movement, with the fingers of your right hand pointing to your left forearm.

This movement is good for your shoulders and protects the energy of the heart.

❹ From here, turn to the left and hold the ball.

❻ Bring the left hand down and around.

❺ Turn to the right, raising the right hand to head height before turning to the front.

4. brush knee and press

With this movement, one hand is deflecting to the side and the other pressing forward at about chest level. The left arm is extended and behind the shoulder, the palm facing up. The right hand is facing down, with the arm bent.

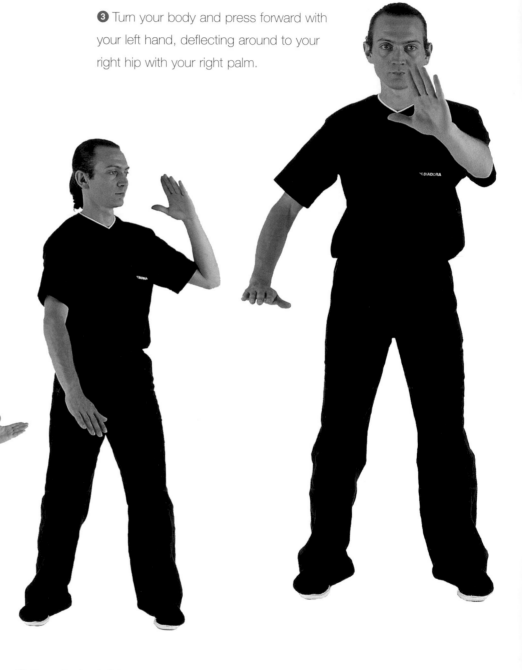

3 Turn your body and press forward with your left hand, deflecting around to your right hip with your right palm.

1 Begin by turning to the left and raising both hands to about shoulder height.

2 Draw in the left hand toward the ear and shoulder and bend the arm. As you do this, lower the right hand to about waist level.

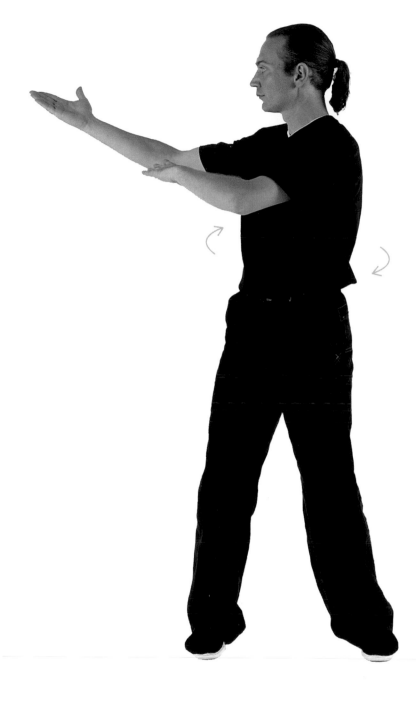

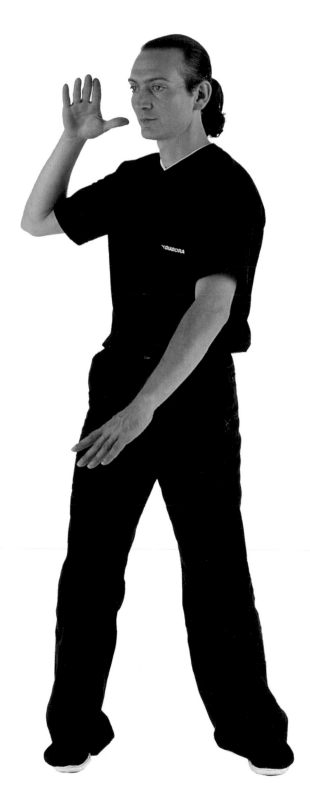

4 The process is repeated for the other side, as shown here.

5. single whip

This is an open, expansive movement that uses the "beak hand." One of the energies here is of separation, as you move the hands apart toward the end of the movement.

❶ Begin by looking at your left hand and turn your body to the left, turning the left palm out.

❷ Start turning to the right.

❸ Raise your right hand as you extend your left and form a crane's beak with the left hand.

❹ Turn to the right. Press forward with your right hand.

5 From here, the movement is repeated on the left side. Turn to the left and open your left hand.

7 Now turn to the left, turning the left hand outward, and press forward.

6 From here, turn to the right and simultaneously raise your left hand as you extend your right arm outward to form a crane's beak, as seen here.

6. cloud hands

This movement is very relaxing and also helps us focus on turning the waist correctly. The name for the movement comes from the symbolism of the hands moving across the body in the way that clouds float across the sky.

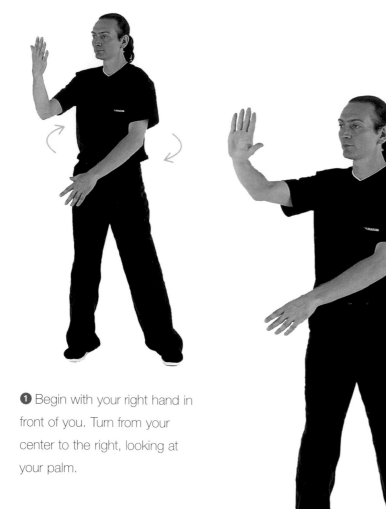

❶ Begin with your right hand in front of you. Turn from your center to the right, looking at your palm.

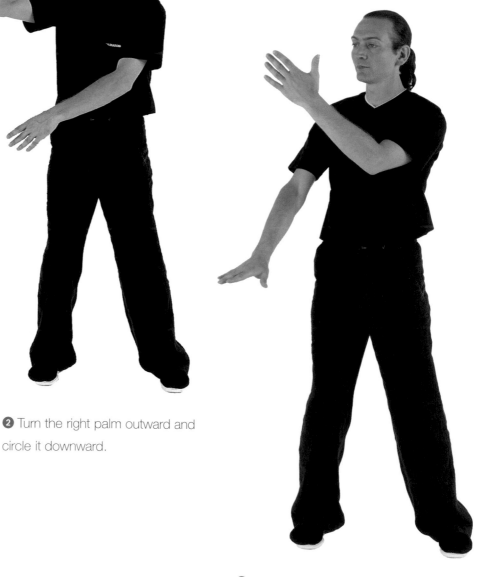

❷ Turn the right palm outward and circle it downward.

❸ At the same time, raise the left palm.

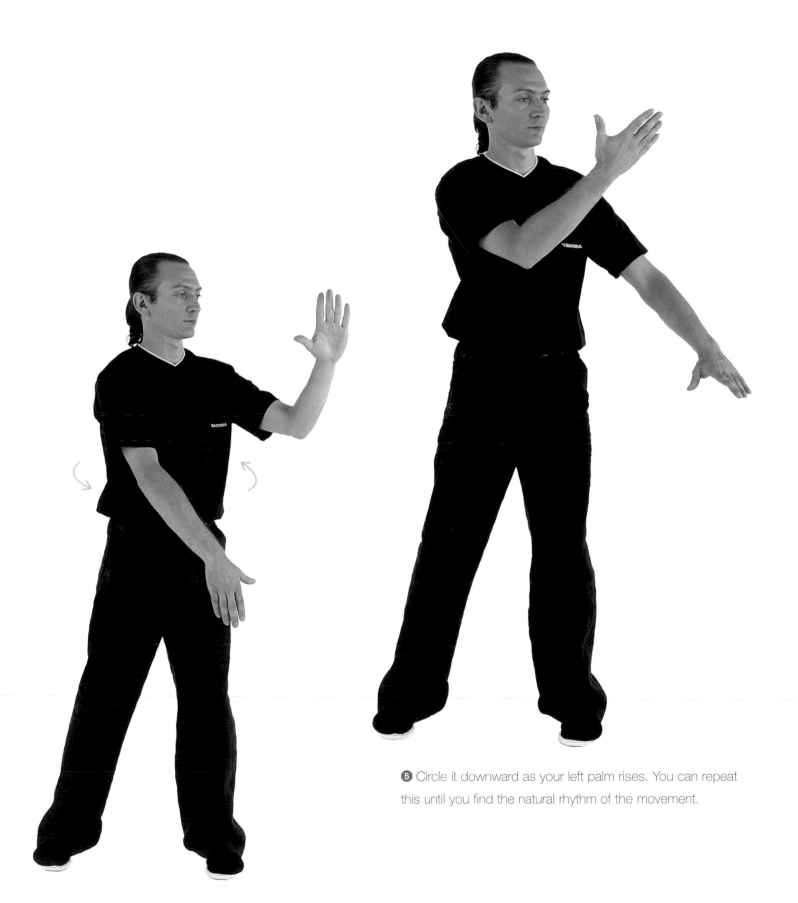

❺ Circle it downward as your left palm rises. You can repeat this until you find the natural rhythm of the movement.

❹ Turn to the left, looking at your palm. Now turn it outward.

7. grasp the bird's tail

This is really four movements in one: Ward Off, Roll Back, Press, and Push (see "The Eight Energies of Tai Chi," pages 42–45). In the photos, a side view is used to make it easier to follow.

ward off (peng)

This is an upward, rounded, outward-expanding movement known as *Peng* in Chinese. It is the first of the Eight Energies of tai chi.

❶ Begin by holding a ball to the left.

❷ Turn to the front, raising the right arm and moving it slightly outward so the whole arm is rounded and at chest height. The left palm presses gently downward to hip height.

1   2   3   4   5   6   7   8   9   10

roll back (lu)

This is an inward, absorbing movement, which turns to the side. Known as *Lu* in Chinese, it is representative of the second tai chi energy.

❶ Turn the right palm outward and forward, with the left palm turned upward, as if to grab an incoming arm at the wrist and elbow.

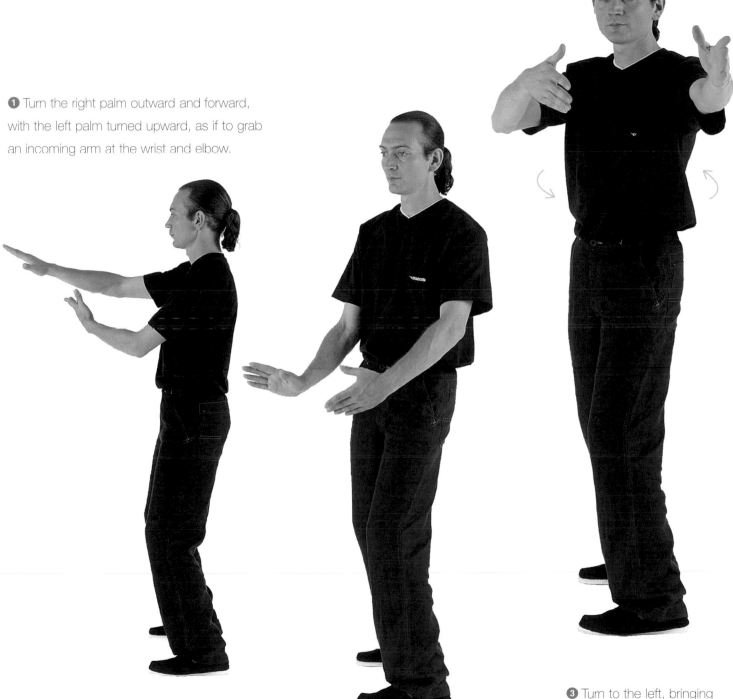

❸ Turn to the left, bringing the palms out to the side.

❷ Draw the palms inward and downward, turning your hips at the same time.

press (ji)

This is known as *Ji* in Chinese and is the third tai chi energy. It is characterized by a straight-ahead force.

❶ From the end of Roll Back, raise the palms in a circular movement, with the left palm making a larger circle than the right. Turn to the front, bringing the palms together.

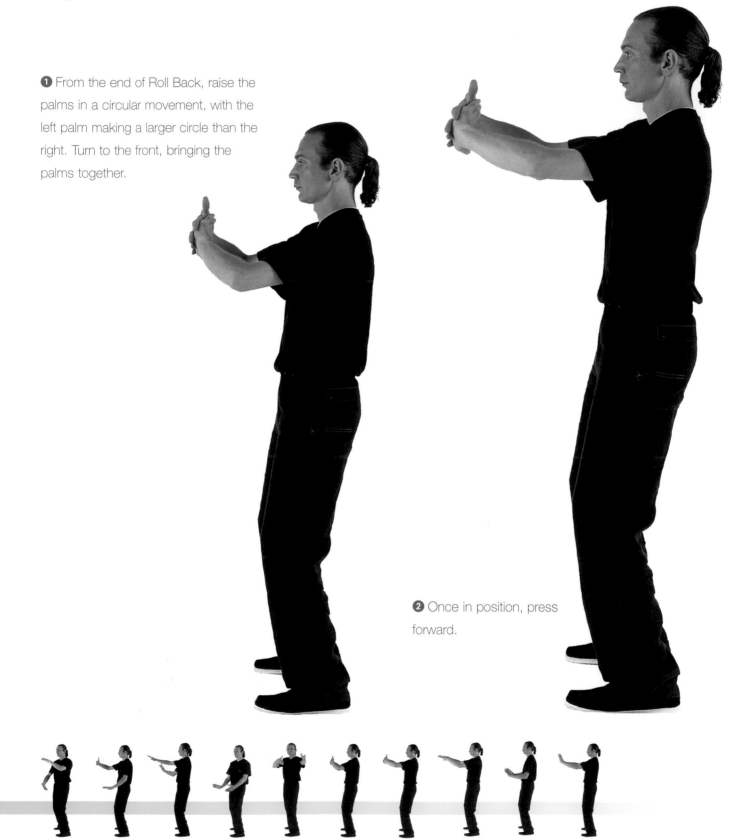

❷ Once in position, press forward.

1   2   3   4   5   6   7   8   9   10

push (an)

This is known as *An* in Chinese and is the fourth of the Eight Energies. It is a downward movement followed by an upward and outward push.

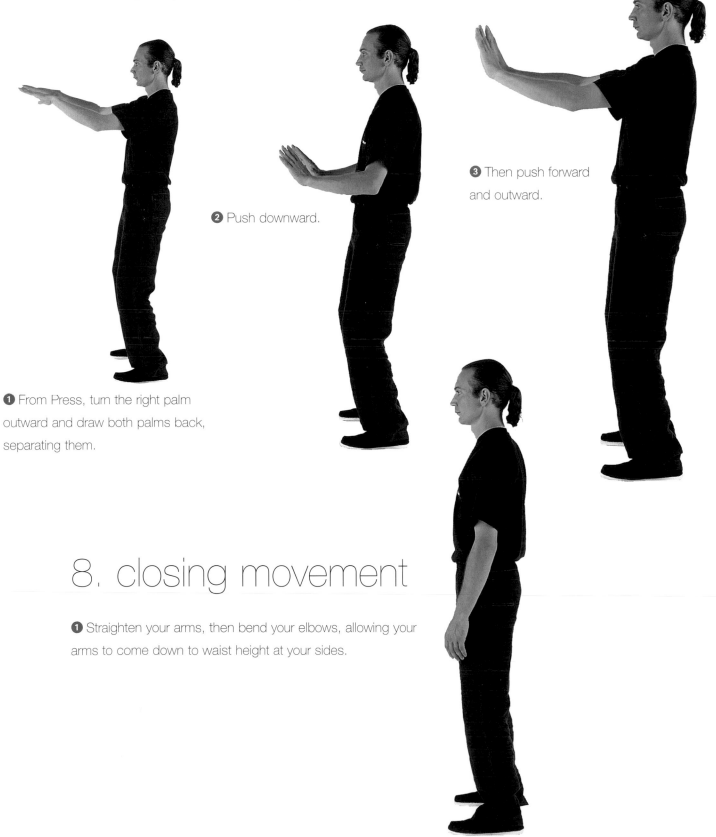

❷ Push downward.

❸ Then push forward and outward.

❶ From Press, turn the right palm outward and draw both palms back, separating them.

8. closing movement

❶ Straighten your arms, then bend your elbows, allowing your arms to come down to waist height at your sides.

The movement is rooted in the feet, developed in the legs, directed by the waist, and expressed through the hands and fingers. From the feet to the legs to the waist should be one unbroken chi flow.

Tai Chi Classics

tai chi footwork

tai chi footwork **using mirror-image postures**

These exercises are designed to give you a good grounding in the basic footwork needed for form practice. The latter exercises will also help you familiarize yourself with combining upper and lower body movements in a unified whole.

The finished stance within these exercises is known as the Bow Stance. This stance occurs throughout the form and it is essential that you become proficient in moving from one Bow Stance to another in order to make any progress with learning a form.

The initial movement (mirror image using Bow Stance) will teach you how to move like a cat, i.e., when you place your foot, there is no weight in it (it remains empty). There are no sudden movements; all the postures should be done in a relaxed way, with a feeling of fluidity. Your balance will improve through doing these exercises as you carefully transfer your weight from one leg to another. Footwork also helps strengthen your legs without impacting your joints.

When you start to do the movements using the upper body, the emphasis changes as more coordination is needed. Without familiarizing yourself with the footwork first, the complex moves needed would be a real struggle. This focus on footwork working in synergy with upper-body movement is a recurring theme within tai chi. It is therefore essential that you complete these exercises before attempting to learn the form.

right: Bow Stance is one of the stances essential to the footwork of tai chi.

mirror image **bow stance**

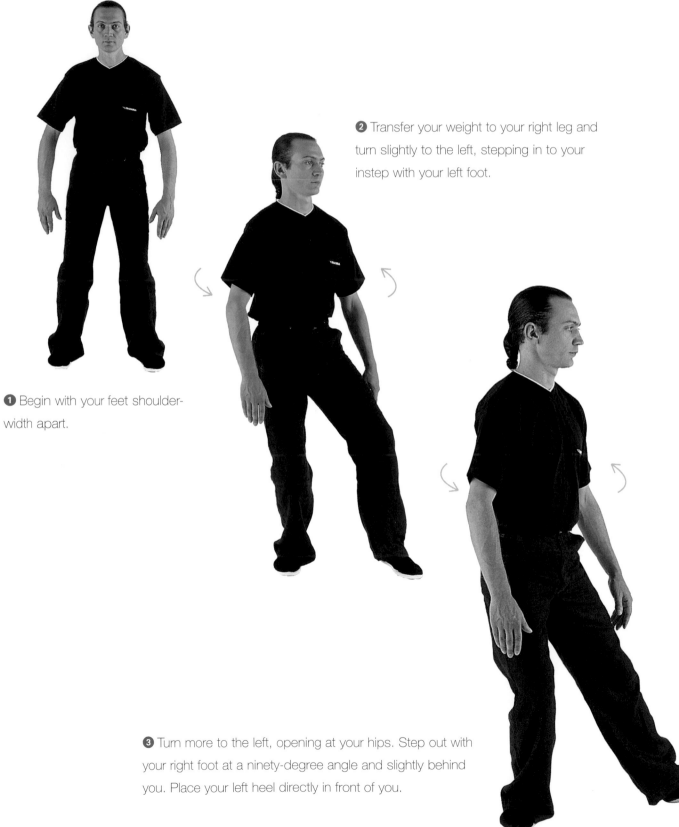

❷ Transfer your weight to your right leg and turn slightly to the left, stepping in to your instep with your left foot.

❶ Begin with your feet shoulder-width apart.

❸ Turn more to the left, opening at your hips. Step out with your right foot at a ninety-degree angle and slightly behind you. Place your left heel directly in front of you.

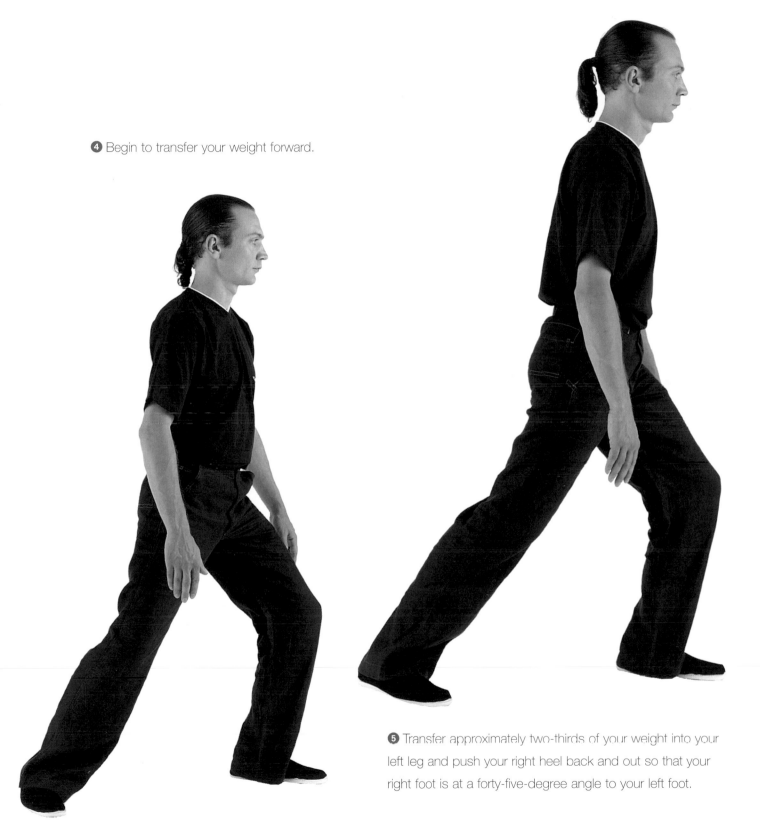

④ Begin to transfer your weight forward.

⑤ Transfer approximately two-thirds of your weight into your left leg and push your right heel back and out so that your right foot is at a forty-five-degree angle to your left foot.

right-sided **bow stance**

From here, we are going to turn 180 degrees to the right to end up in a right-sided Bow Stance.

❶ From the left Bow Stance, transfer all your weight to your right leg.

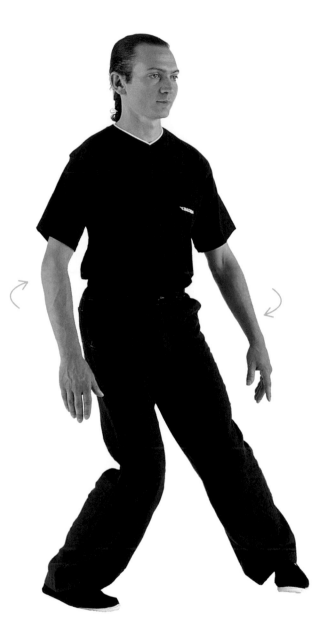

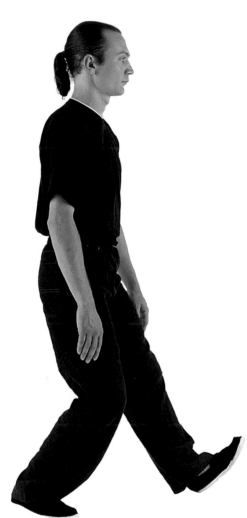

❷ Turn your body and left foot about ninety degrees to the right.

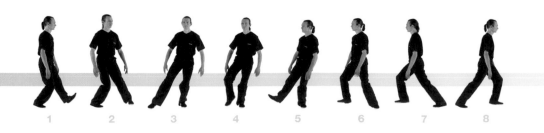

1   2   3   4   5   6   7   8

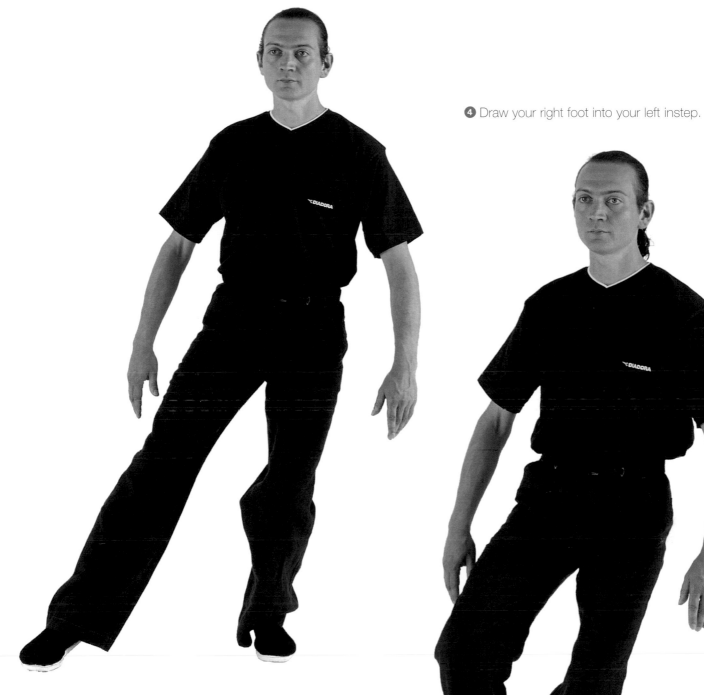

4 Draw your right foot into your left instep.

3 Transfer all your weight to your left leg, maintaining your posture without raising the height of the stance.

6 Place your right foot on the ground heel-first while keeping the weight on the back foot. Begin to transfer your weight forward and turn your waist and hips so your body is also facing forward.

5 Step out and forward, with your right foot in an arc.

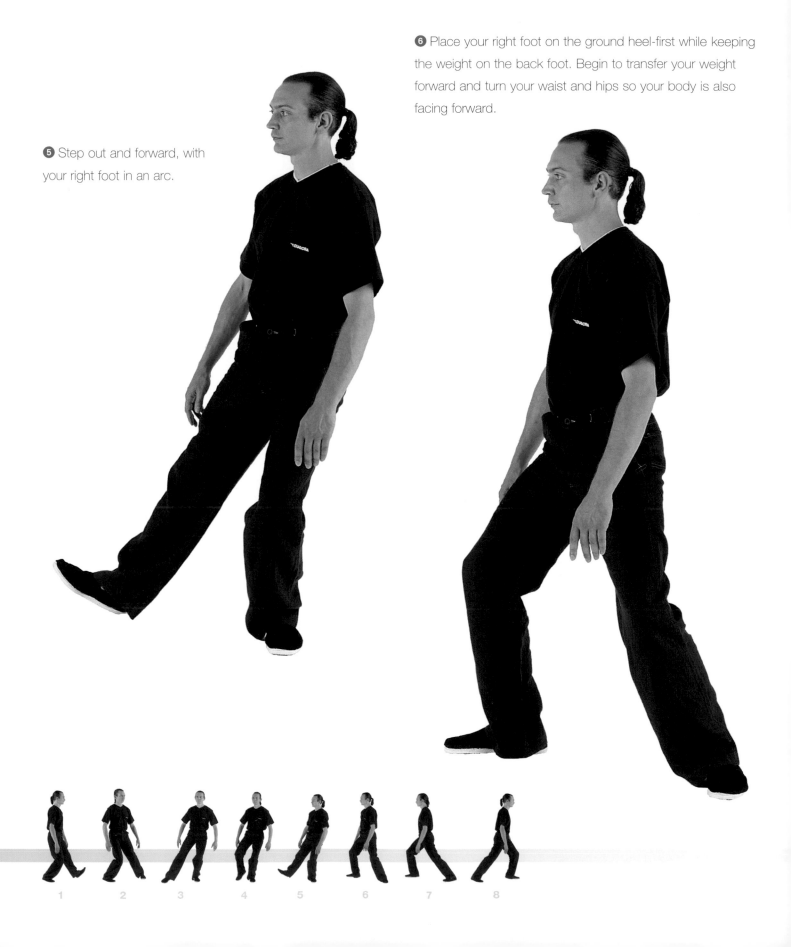

1   2   3   4   5   6   7   8

This exercise should be done carefully and slowly. All the points of posture still apply, so remember to keep your back straight and relaxed. There is a saying in tai chi that motion is rooted in the feet, transmitted through the legs, directed by the waist, and manifested in the fingers. This can, in part, be seen here and in the next few exercises, where we use the hand movements of Parting the Wild Horse's Mane and Brush Knee and Press.

7 Continue by adjusting your back heel. You are now in a right-sided Bow Stance.

8 Repeat by transferring your weight back, turning ninety degrees to the left, shifting your weight onto the right leg, and stepping in to the right instep with the left foot. Step forward and out with the left foot, at ninety degrees to your right foot, and shift your weight forward into a left-sided Bow Stance. Repeat the whole sequence until you are familiar with it and your movement begins to flow.

mirror image **parting the wild horse's mane**

This exercise helps promote coordination. The footwork here is the same as before.

1 Begin as if you have finished the first movement.

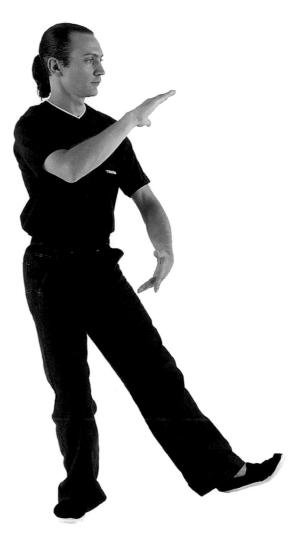

2 Transfer your weight to your right leg and begin to turn slightly to the left. Draw your left foot into the instep, raise your right hand, and form an imaginary ball, as pictured at right.

3 Step out as in the previous exercise.

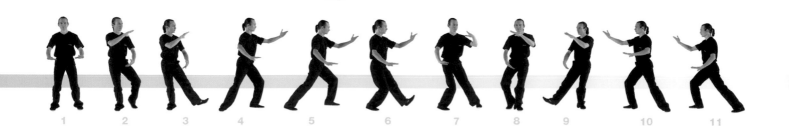

1   2   3   4   5   6   7   8   9   10   11

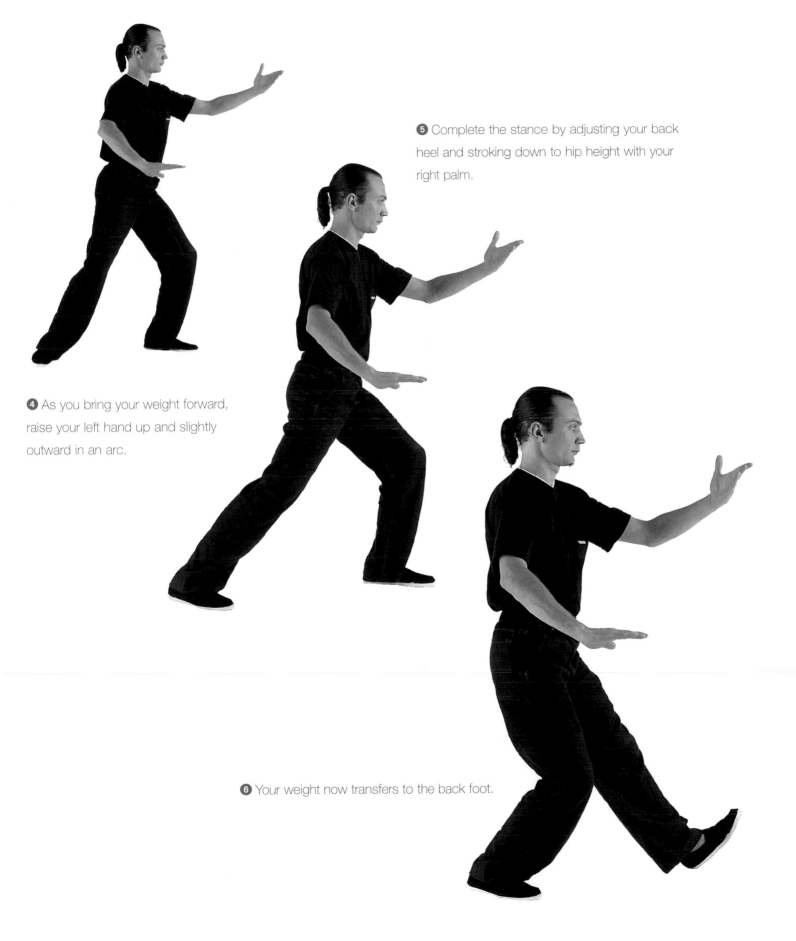

5 Complete the stance by adjusting your back heel and stroking down to hip height with your right palm.

4 As you bring your weight forward, raise your left hand up and slightly outward in an arc.

6 Your weight now transfers to the back foot.

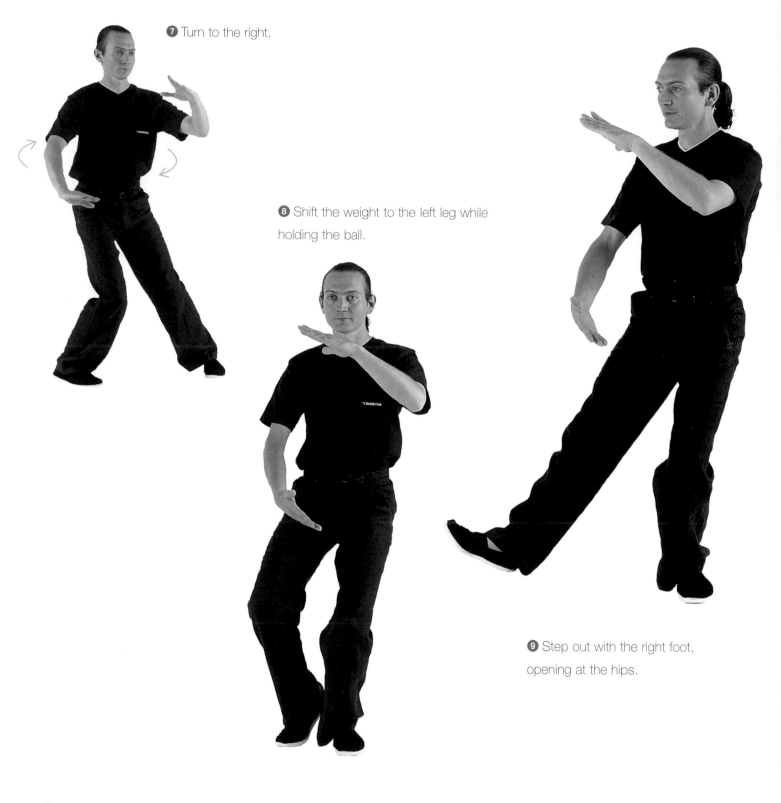

❼ Turn to the right.

❽ Shift the weight to the left leg while holding the ball.

❾ Step out with the right foot, opening at the hips.

1   2   3   4   5   6   7   8   9   10   11

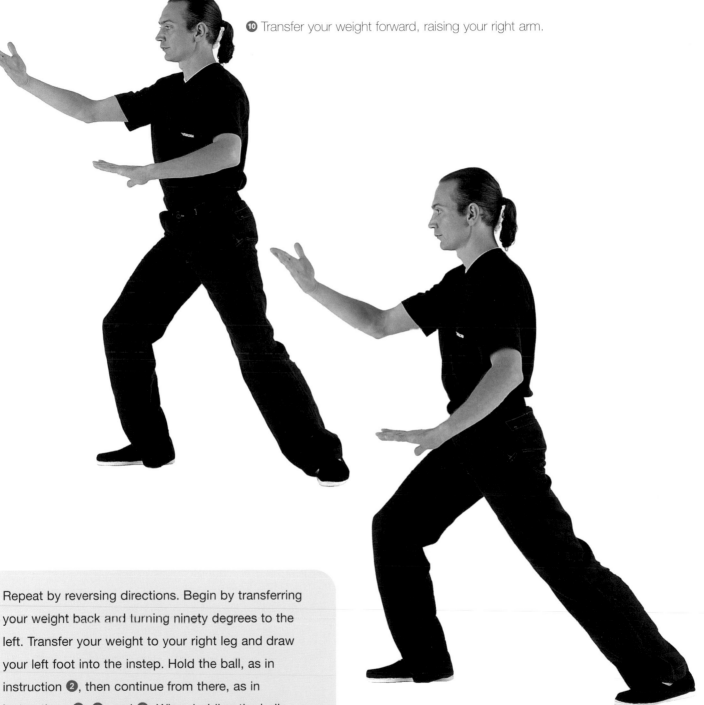

⓾ Transfer your weight forward, raising your right arm.

Repeat by reversing directions. Begin by transferring your weight back and turning ninety degrees to the left. Transfer your weight to your right leg and draw your left foot into the instep. Hold the ball, as in instruction ➋, then continue from there, as in instructions ➌, ➍, and ➎. When holding the ball, your elbows should be relaxed and facing downward.

⓫ Stroke down with your left palm as you adjust your left heel.

mirror image   **brush knee and press**

Here the footwork of the tai chi walk is combined with the upper-body movement Brush Knee and Press. Timing and coordination are key elements here.

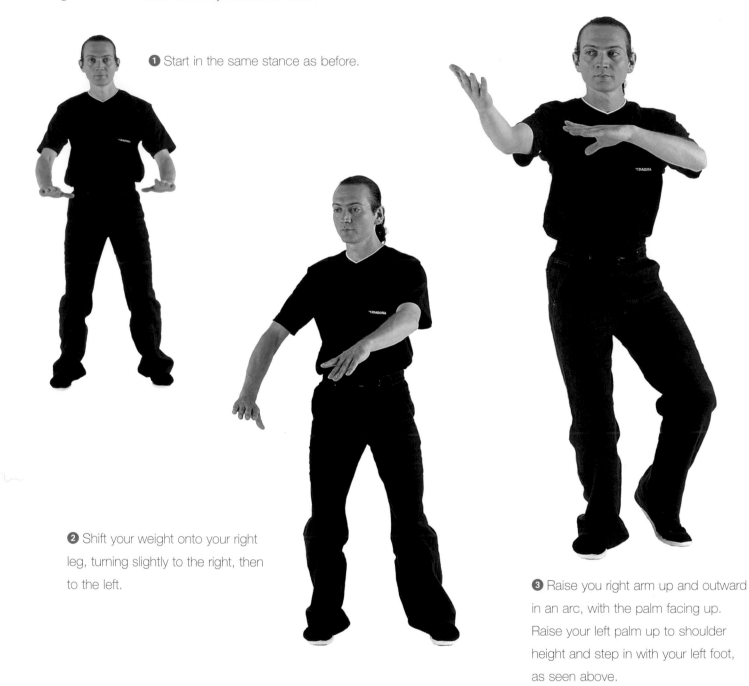

❶ Start in the same stance as before.

❷ Shift your weight onto your right leg, turning slightly to the right, then to the left.

❸ Raise you right arm up and outward in an arc, with the palm facing up. Raise your left palm up to shoulder height and step in with your left foot, as seen above.

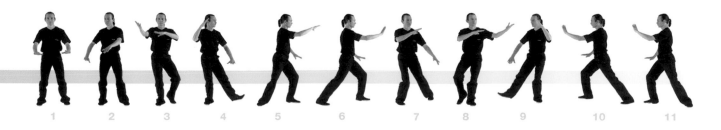

1   2   3   4   5   6   7   8   9   10   11

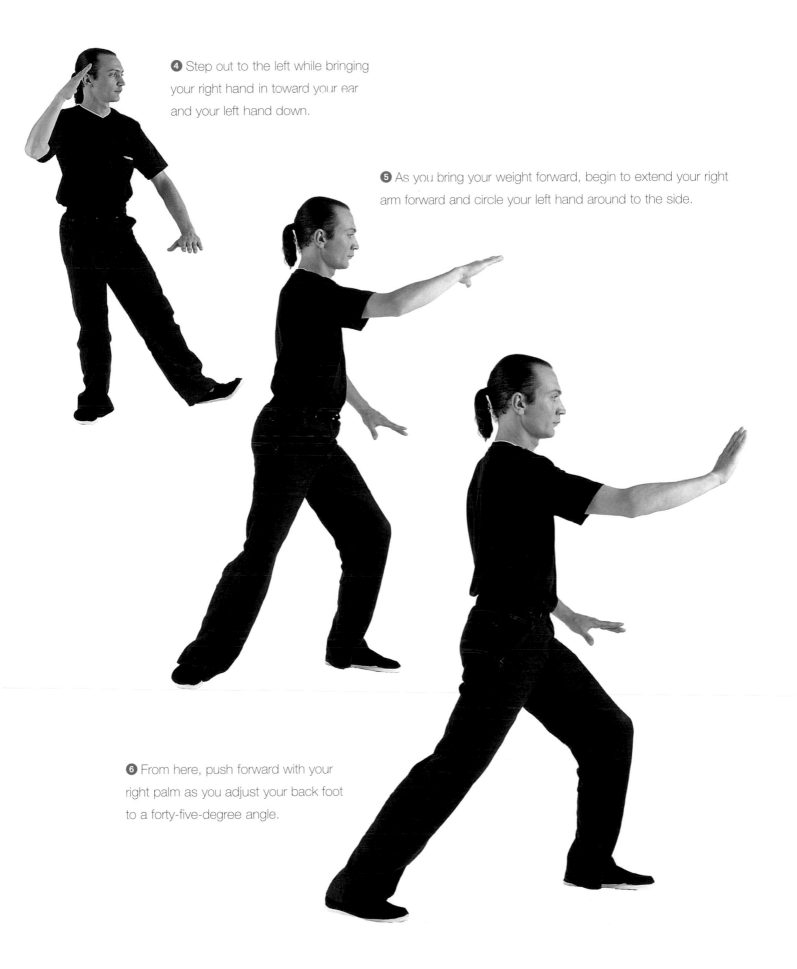

❹ Step out to the left while bringing your right hand in toward your ear and your left hand down.

❺ As you bring your weight forward, begin to extend your right arm forward and circle your left hand around to the side.

❻ From here, push forward with your right palm as you adjust your back foot to a forty-five-degree angle.

❼ From here, transfer your weight back and hook your left foot around ninety degrees.

❽ Transfer your weight onto your left leg and raise your left hand to shoulder height as you bring your right foot into your left instep.

❾ Step out with your right foot to a ninety-degree angle while bringing your left hand in toward your ear and your right hand down.

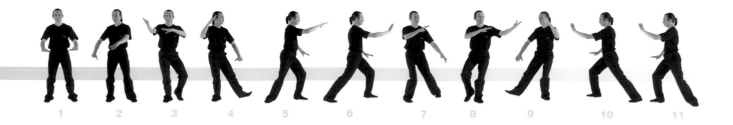

1   2   3   4   5   6   7   8   9   10   11

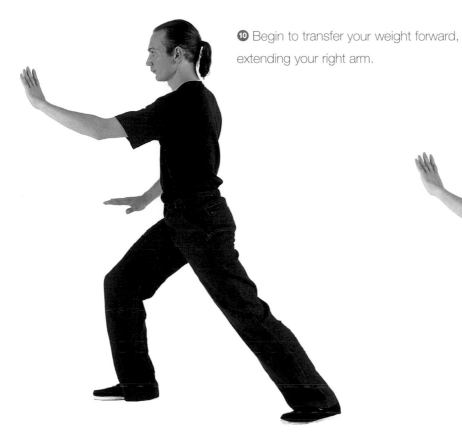

⑩ Begin to transfer your weight forward, extending your right arm.

⑪ Press forward with your right palm and adjust your back heel on the ball of the foot to a forty-five-degree angle.

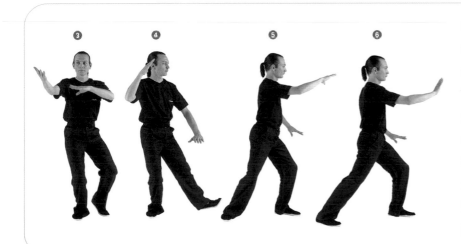

From here, the direction is reversed. Begin by transferring your weight back and turn ninety degrees to the left while hooking your right foot around. Transfer your weight to your right leg and begin to raise your left hand to shoulder height, as in ❸. The sequence then follows the same pattern as ❹ to ❻. Repeat until your movements gradually become more proficient and smooth. (When stepping out, as in ❹ and ❾, remember to coordinate the step with the simultaneous movements of both arms.)

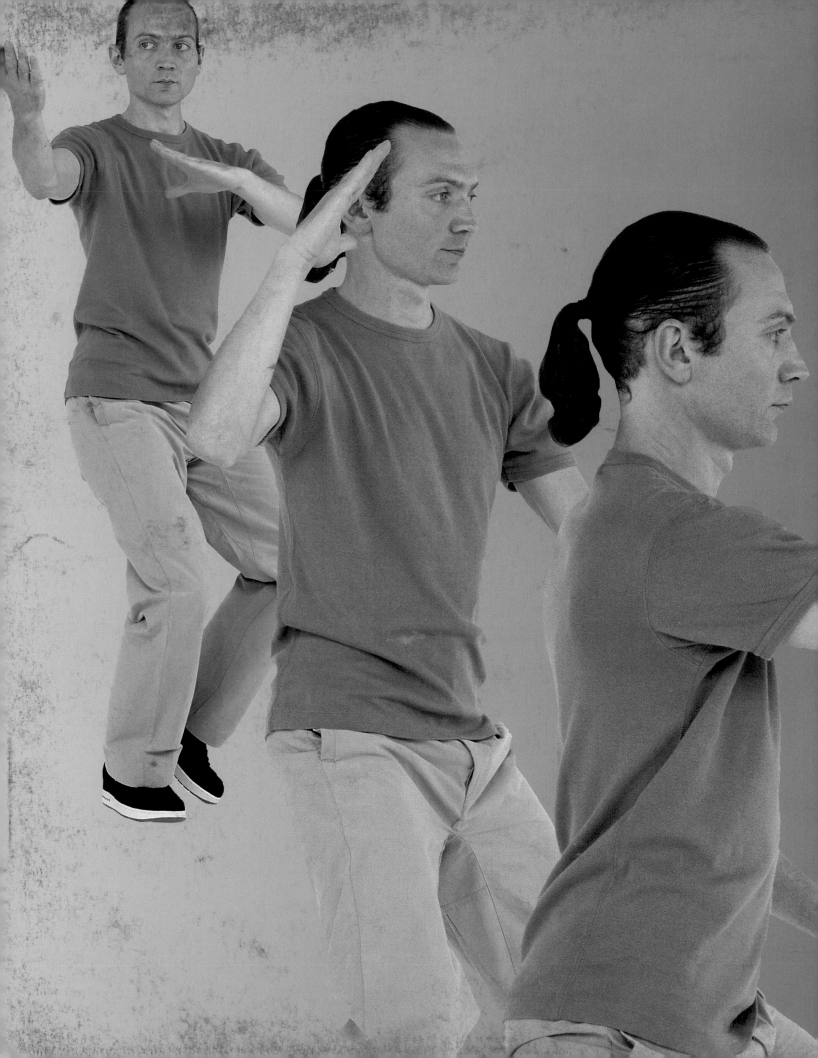

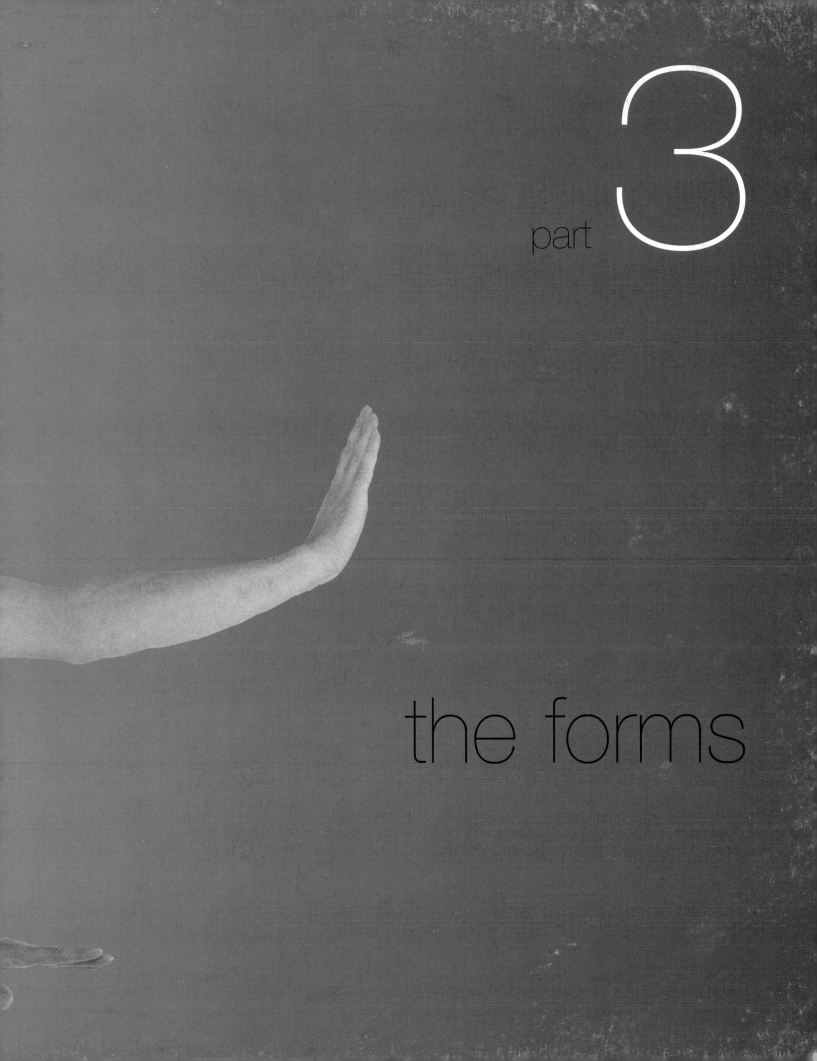

part 3

the forms

Always remember that when one part moves, all parts move; when one part is still, all parts are still.

Tai Chi Classics

the eight-posture simplified yang style form

tai chi forms

There are many tai chi forms taught throughout the world. Within each style there can be many variations and interpretations. However, what unites tai chi styles and forms are the common principles involved and the underlying philosophy.

The two tai chi forms presented in this book are designed to give the beginner and intermediate student a form that can be learned relatively easily and that can become the basis of a good foundation for practice and development. For practitioners with previous experience, they will give an insight into other ways of working and might provide further ideas to improve your own studies.

For very experienced practitioners, the forms provide a framework for practice and deepening study, along with Push Hands, Fa Jin, weapons forms, and Da Lu (two-person routines).

One of the most important things about forms is that they give us a framework for practicing correct structure and alignment. Before we can develop the chi vitality or internal power, we need to learn how to align our bodies so that energy can circulate properly. If these alignments are seen as electrical circuits and the chi as electricity, the correct circuitry is essential.

The Eight-Posture Form was devised in 1998 in Beijing and forms part of a structured training syllabus created by the International Wu Shu Federation. The syllabus in its entirety includes:
• Eight-, Sixteen-, and Twenty-four-Posture Simplified Yang Style Tai Chi Chuan
• Thirty-two- and Forty-two-Posture Combined Tai Chi Chuan (Yang, Wu, Chen, and Sun style)
• Sixteen-, Thirty-two-, Thirty-four-, and Forty-two-Posture Tai Chi Jian (Sword)

The Eight-Posture Form is a short sequence by tai chi standards and is very accessible to beginners. It can be learned in a period of a few weeks, which makes it especially attractive, yet all the principles of tai chi are present, as are the benefits.

1. open tai chi

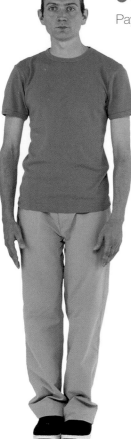

❶ Start with your feet together and your body relaxed. Pay attention to the sensations in your body.

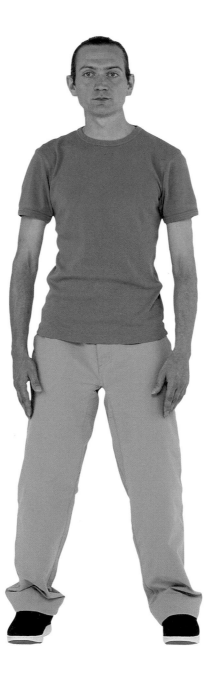

❷ Sink your weight into your right leg and step out with your left foot, to shoulder-width.

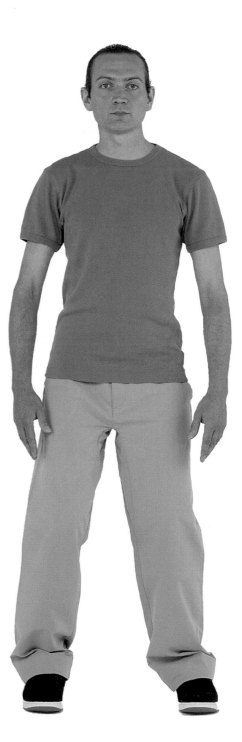

❸ Center your body weight.

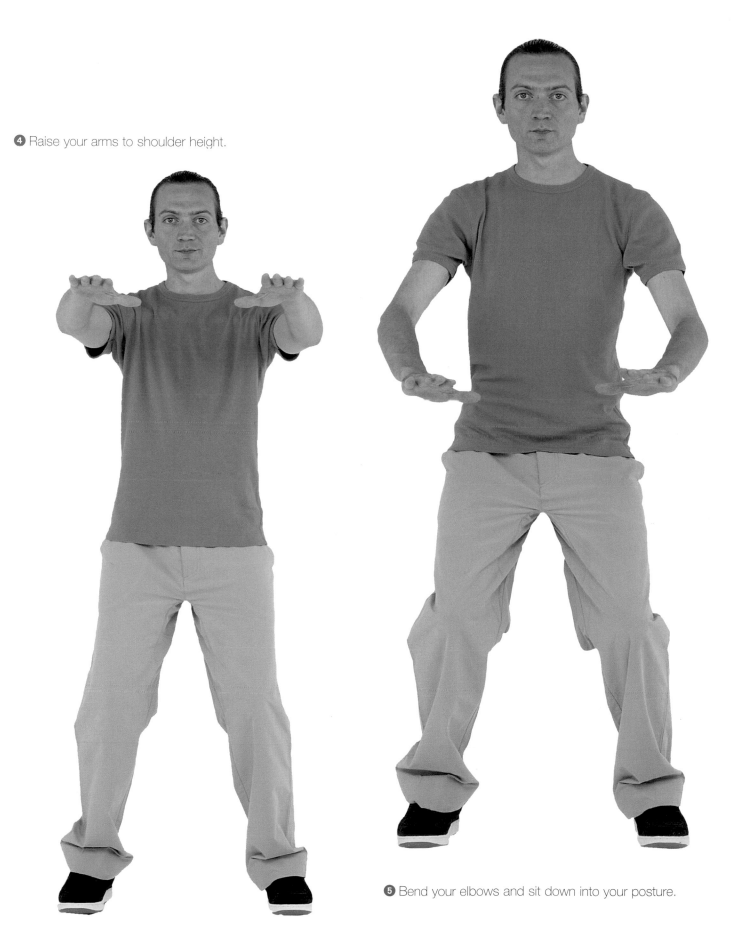

❹ Raise your arms to shoulder height.

❺ Bend your elbows and sit down into your posture.

2. parting the wild horse's mane

From Open Tai Chi, transfer your weight onto your right leg, turning slightly to the right. Turn to the left and raise your right hand to about chest height.

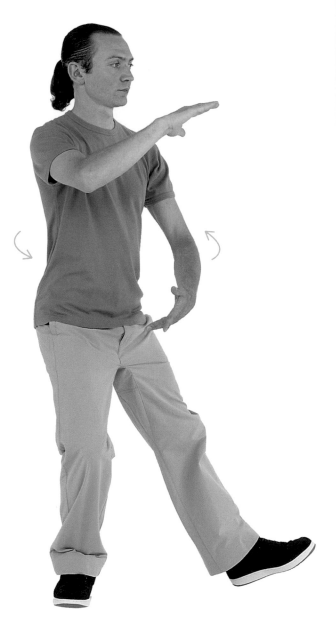

❶ Step in with your left foot to your right instep and hold the ball.

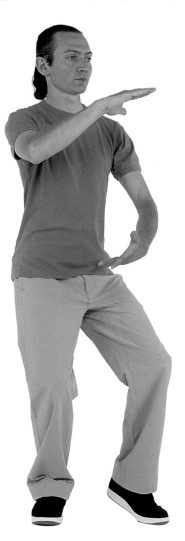

❷ Turn to the left and step out and forward with your left foot. Your left foot should now be at a ninety-degree angle to your right foot.

1   2   3   4   5   6   7   8

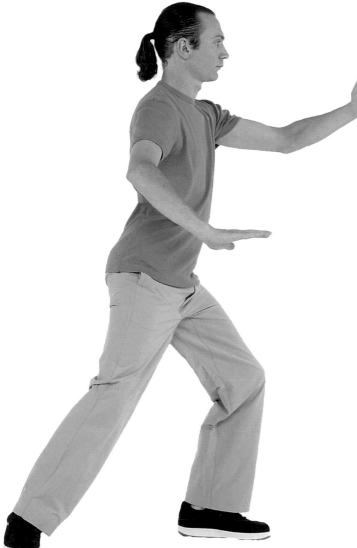

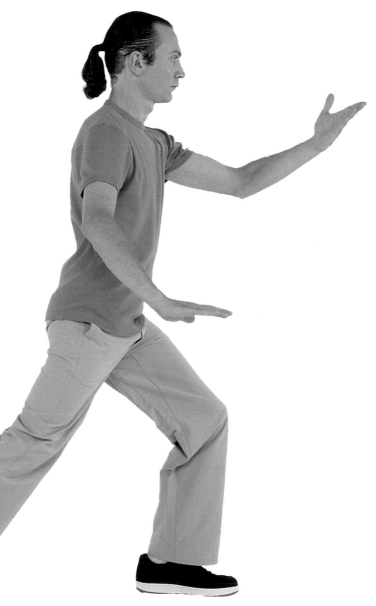

❹ You are now in a left-sided Bow Stance, with two-thirds of your weight on your left leg.

❸ Transfer your weight forward and turn your waist and hips. As you do this, raise the left hand up in an arc and stroke down the inside of your forearm with your right hand. Adjust your back heel to a forty-five-degree angle by pushing it back and turning on the ball of the foot.

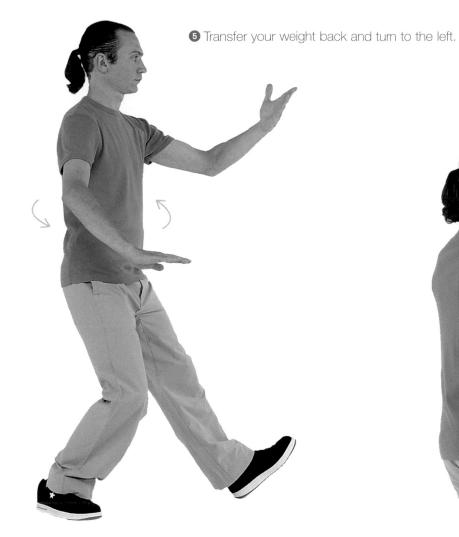

5 Transfer your weight back and turn to the left.

6 Transfer your weight forward and step up with your right foot. Hold the ball, with the left hand on top.

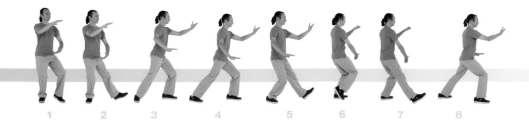

1   2   3   4   5   6   7   8

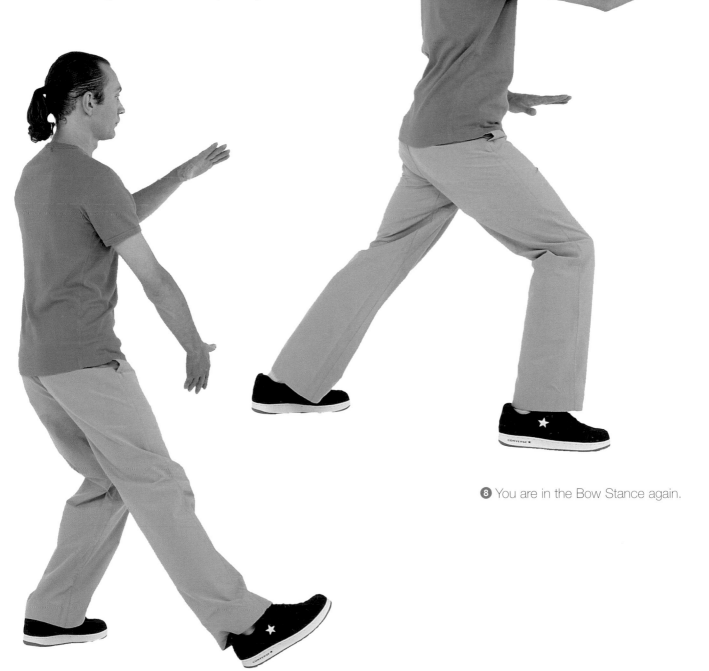

7 Step forward and out with your right foot. Transfer your weight forward and turn your body, raising the right hand in an arc and stroking down to the left hip with your left hand.

8 You are in the Bow Stance again.

3. white crane spreads its wings

White Crane is done in an empty stance, with all the weight ending up on your left leg. (An empty stance is one in which the body's weight falls onto one leg or the other.) The feeling here is open and expansive.

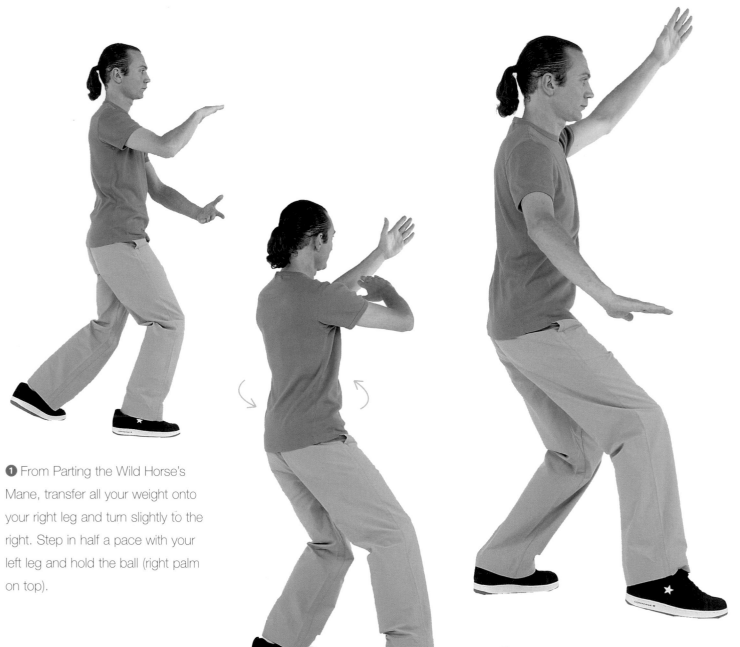

❶ From Parting the Wild Horse's Mane, transfer all your weight onto your right leg and turn slightly to the right. Step in half a pace with your left leg and hold the ball (right palm on top).

❷ Sink your weight into your left leg and turn to the left corner, raising your left hand to about head height. The right palm follows the movement.

❸ Turn to the front and lower the right hand across the body toward the right. Relax and sink into your left leg.

4. brush knee and press

The transition here is the key. The rest of the movement is the same as used for the tai chi Mirror Image exercises (see pages 90–93).

❶ From White Crane, turn to the right and turn your left forearm in so that your left palm is now facing you.

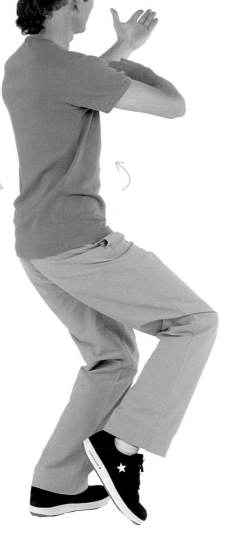

❷ Bring the left palm down, opposite the centerline of your body, and raise your right palm, face up.

❸ Turn to the left and bring the left hand up in an arc behind you. Step in with your right foot and press down with your right hand.

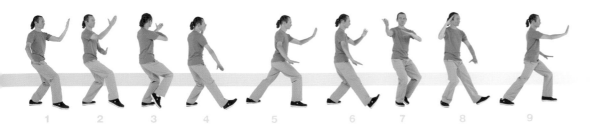

1   2   3   4   5   6   7   8   9

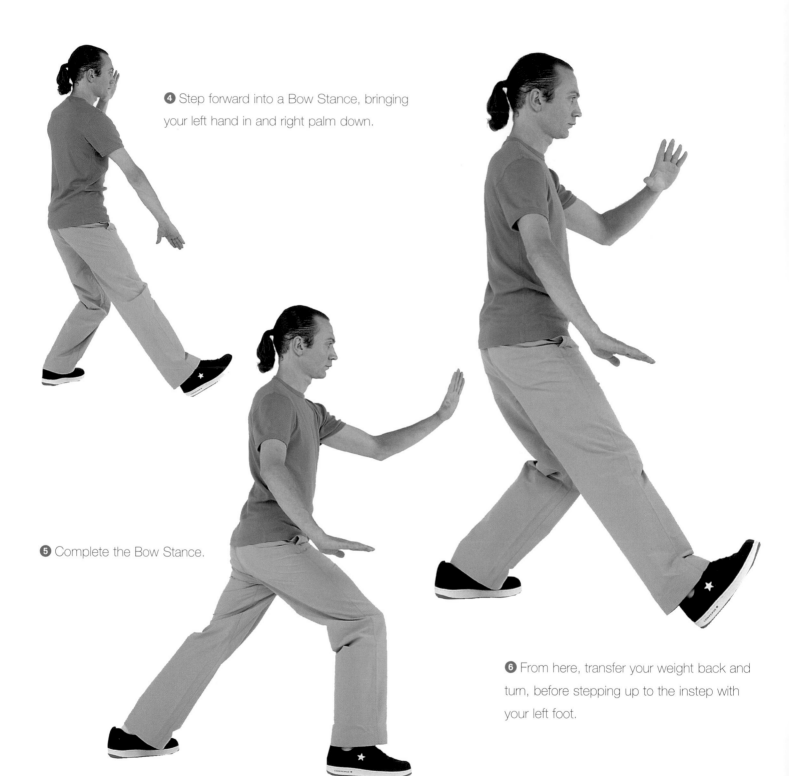

❹ Step forward into a Bow Stance, bringing your left hand in and right palm down.

❺ Complete the Bow Stance.

❻ From here, transfer your weight back and turn, before stepping up to the instep with your left foot.

1   2   3   4   5   6   7   8   9

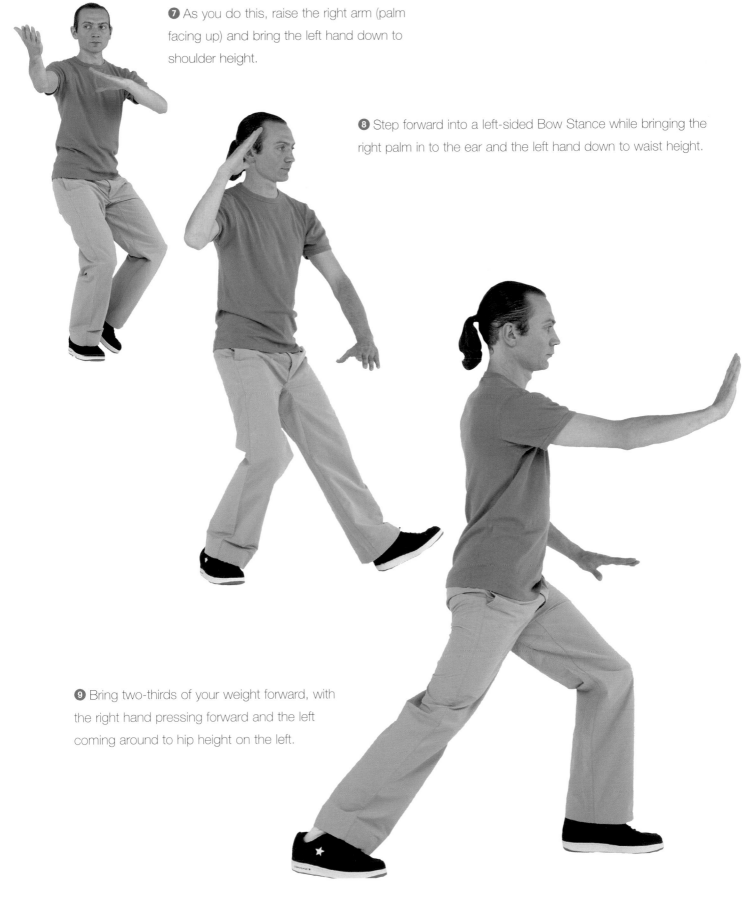

7 As you do this, raise the right arm (palm facing up) and bring the left hand down to shoulder height.

8 Step forward into a left-sided Bow Stance while bringing the right palm in to the ear and the left hand down to waist height.

9 Bring two-thirds of your weight forward, with the right hand pressing forward and the left coming around to hip height on the left.

5. single whip

Here we turn 180 degrees into a right-sided Bow Stance, using the upper-body movement we used before.

❶ From Parting the Wild Horse's Mane, transfer all your weight back onto your right leg and turn to the right, hooking your left foot around ninety degrees.

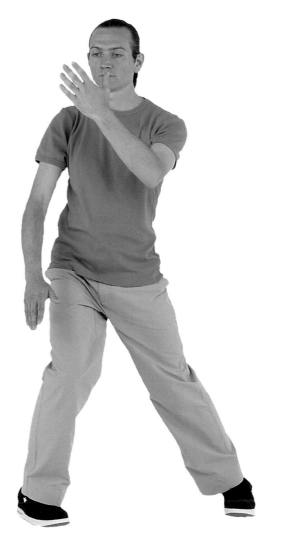

❷ Circle the right palm down and the left palm up.

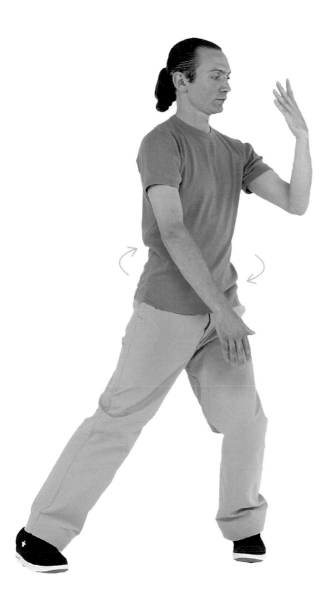

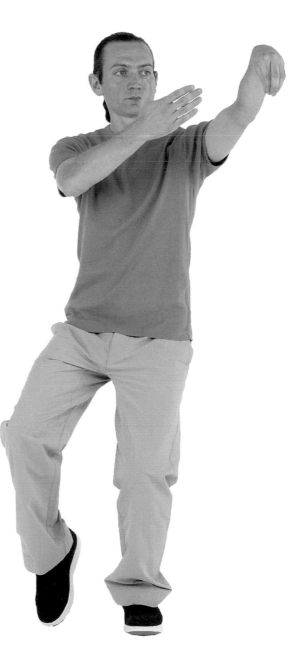

❸ Shift your weight onto your left leg. Turn slightly to the right. From here, push the left hand outward and raise your right hand.

❹ Step in to your left instep and form a crane's beak (wrist bent and all fingers around your thumb) with your left hand, as shown.

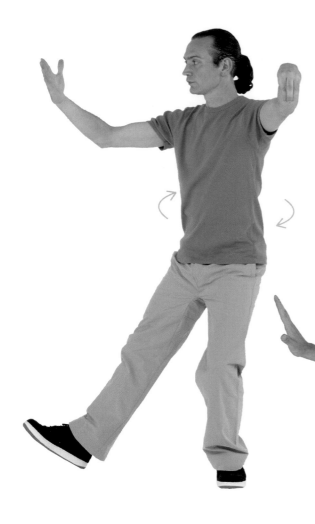

5 Turn and step out to the right with the right foot and transfer two-thirds of your weight to your right leg.

6 Turn the right forearm and press forward with the right palm as you push your left heel back to form a right-sided Bow Stance.

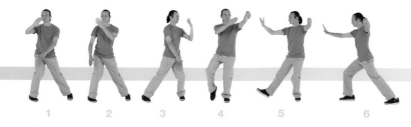

1   2   3   4   5   6

6. cloud hands

With Cloud Hands, the stances are with the feet parallel and the weight on one leg or the other. After the transition from Single Whip, the hand movements are done as in the upper-body movements. The key with Cloud Hands is to simultaneously swap the relative positions of the hands as you step in or out. In total, the pattern is repeated three times. There are three steps in and two steps out.

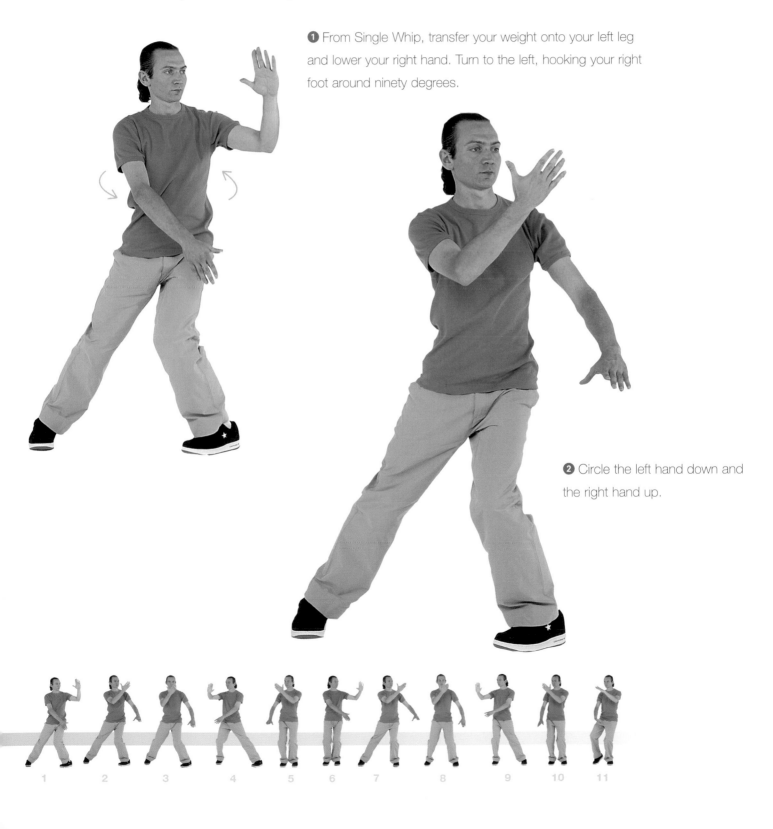

❶ From Single Whip, transfer your weight onto your left leg and lower your right hand. Turn to the left, hooking your right foot around ninety degrees.

❷ Circle the left hand down and the right hand up.

1   2   3   4   5   6   7   8   9   10   11

3 Transfer your weight onto your right leg, turning your waist to the right.

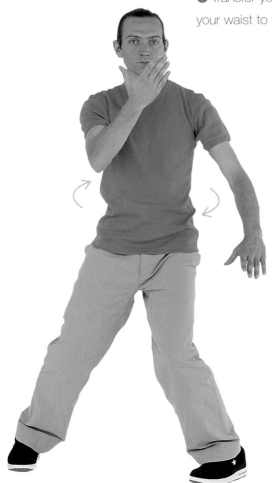

4 Turn your right palm and circle it down as you step in with your left foot to create a parallel stance.

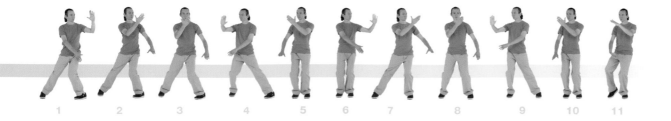

1   2   3   4   5   6   7   8   9   10   11

5 As you do this, raise your left hand. Transfer your weight onto your left leg and turn to the left.

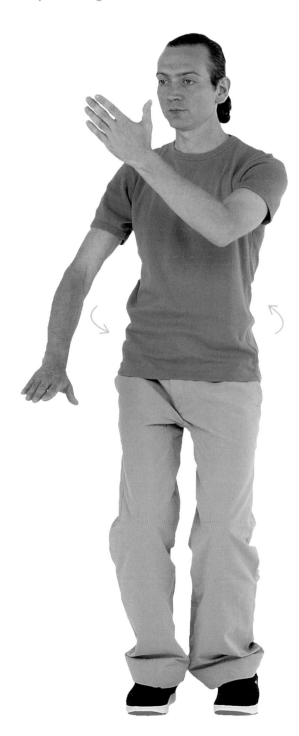

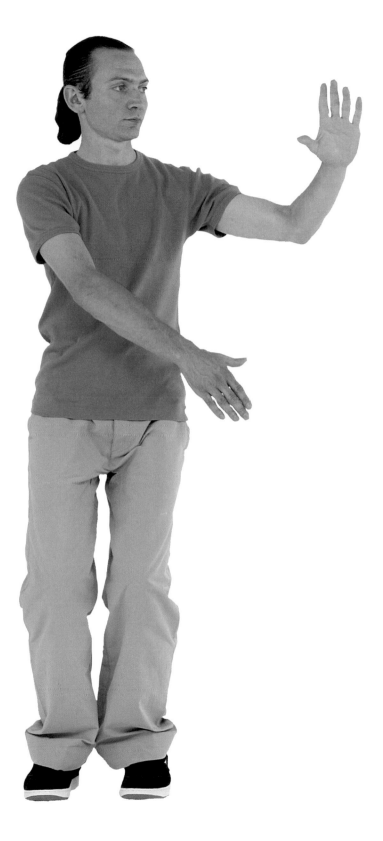

6 Turn the left palm and bring it down in a circle.

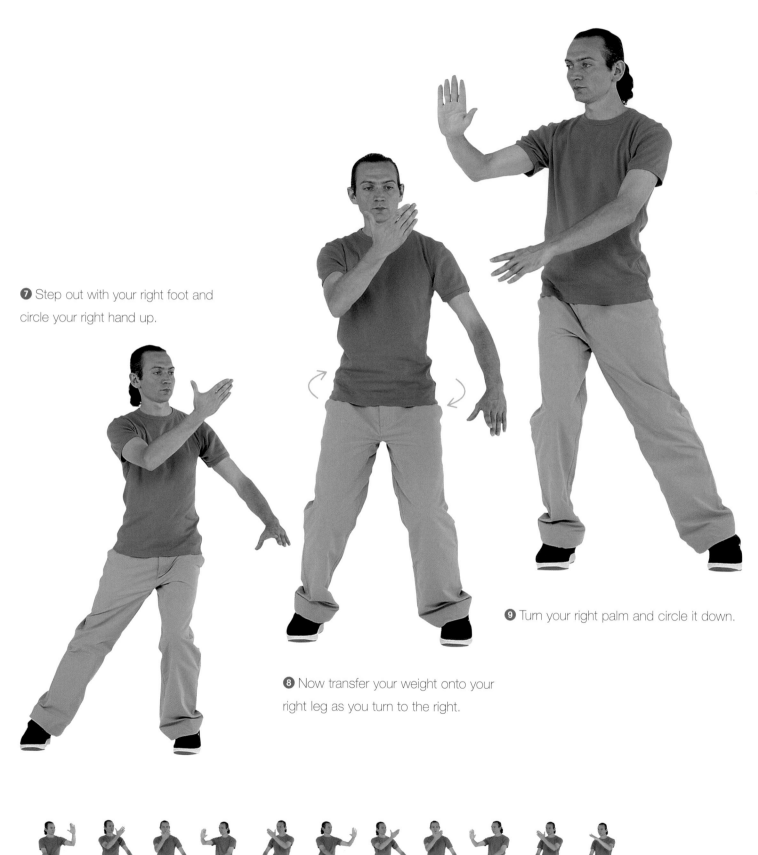

❼ Step out with your right foot and circle your right hand up.

❽ Now transfer your weight onto your right leg as you turn to the right.

❾ Turn your right palm and circle it down.

1   2   3   4   5   6   7   8   9   10   11

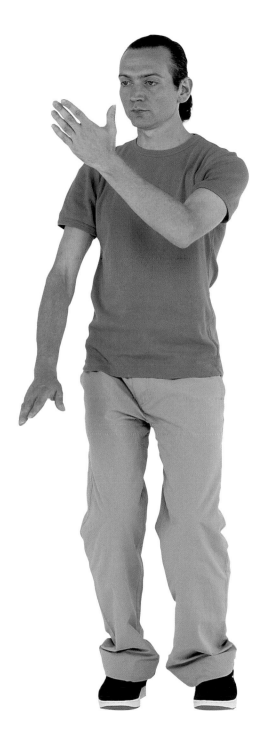

10 Bring your left palm up and step in with your left foot.

11 Repeat again to the left, then the right, and as you step in with your left leg and raise your left hand, sink the weight into your left leg and hold the ball.

7. grasp the bird's tail

1 Step out to form a right-sided Bow Stance. As you turn to the right, raise your right arm and press down with your left.

2 As you shift two-thirds of your weight forward, press forward slightly with the right arm. Adjust your back heel to forty-five degrees. This is Ward Off.

3 From here, turn slightly to the right and turn your right and left hands, as shown.

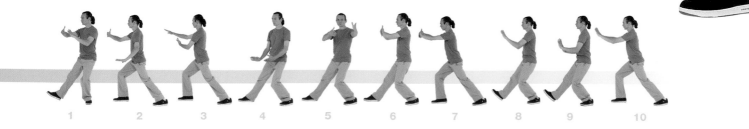

1   2   3   4   5   6   7   8   9   10

4 As if grabbing an elbow and wrist, draw in toward you (shifting your weight onto your back leg) and to the side, turning your waist and hips. This is Roll Back.

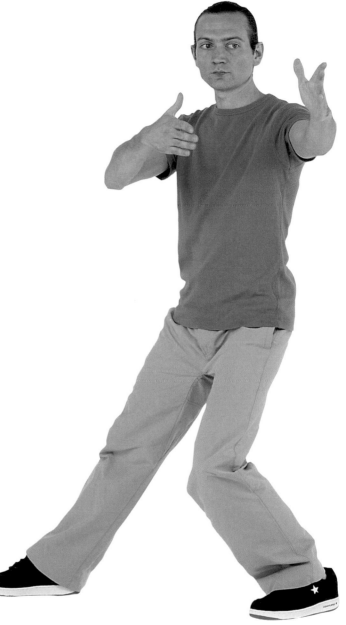

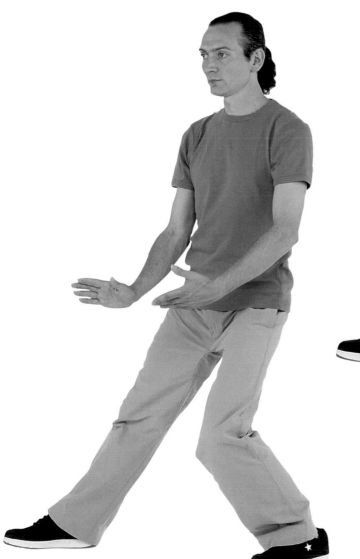

5 Circle your palms to the side and up, as shown (the left hand makes a larger circle). Turn back to face the front.

7 Press forward, bringing two-thirds of your weight forward and into a Bow Stance. This is Press.

8 From here, turn your right hand outward and shift your weight back, separating your hands.

6 Place your left hand inside your right.

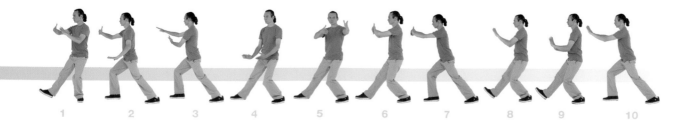

1   2   3   4   5   6   7   8   9   10

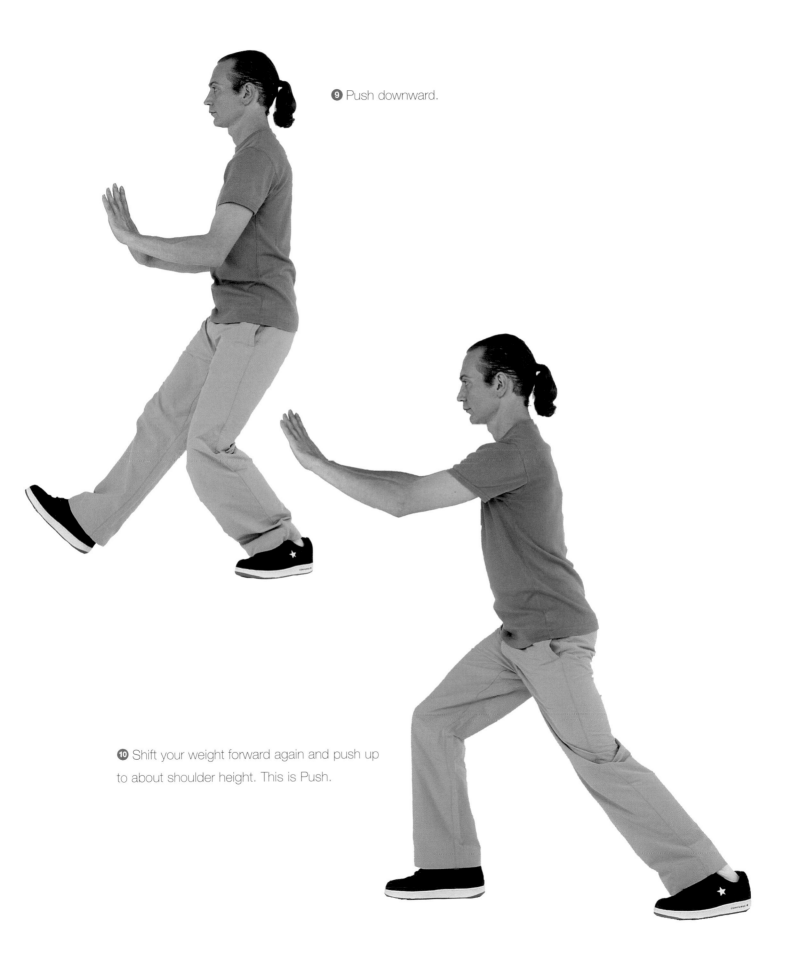

9 Push downward.

10 Shift your weight forward again and push up
to about shoulder height. This is Push.

8. close

❶ Center your body weight and turn to the left, hooking your right foot around ninety degrees.

❷ Turn your left foot around ninety degrees and bring two-thirds of your weight into it while opening outward through the arms and hands.

❸ Shift your weight back onto your right leg.

❺ Come out of the seated posture into an ordinary standing position, bringing your arms and palms down to the sides of your body as you do so.

❻ Step in with your left foot. The sequence is finished.

❹ Step in with your left foot to a shoulder's width.

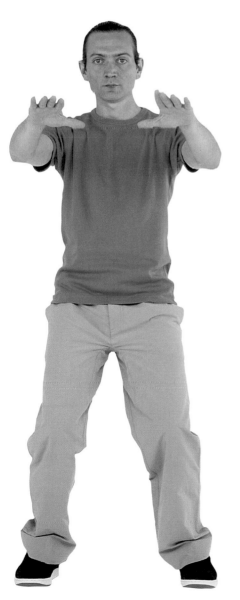

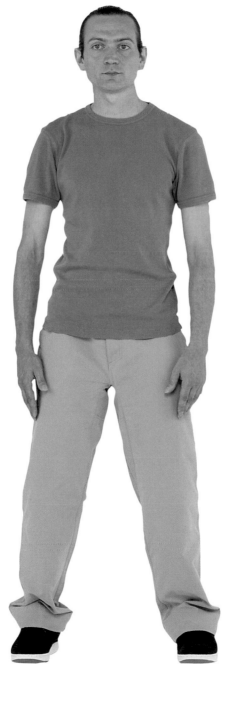

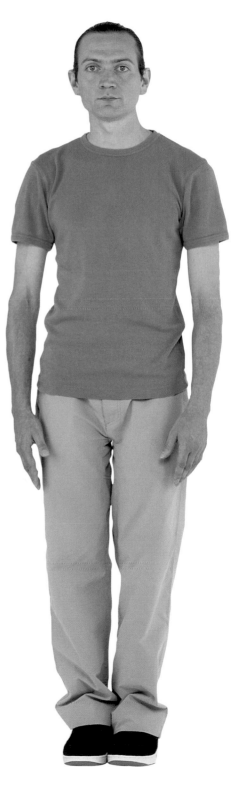

Seek the straight from the curved. Store energy first, and then issue it. To withdraw is to attack and to attack is to withdraw.

Tai Chi Classics

the sixteen-posture form

the sixteen-posture form

This form is more challenging and has more complex movements and demanding postures. Some of the movements are as they appear in the Eight-Posture Form, and some have been reversed. There are nine new movements in this form, so take your time with these. Repeat them at least twelve times to become familiar with them.

caution: Snake Creeps Down is a fairly demanding movement, so some stretches may be necessary beforehand. Adapt this movement if you find it too hard to sink low down. You should only work within your limits.

1. open tai chi

This is exactly the same as it appears in the Eight-Posture Form.

❶ Start with your feet together and your body relaxed. Pay attention to the sensations in your body.

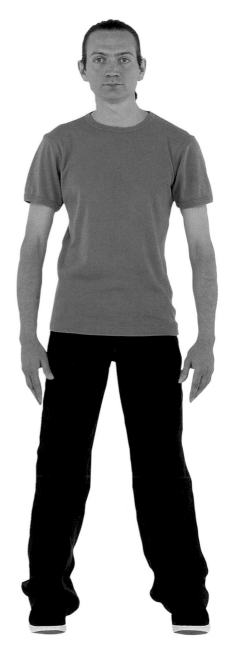

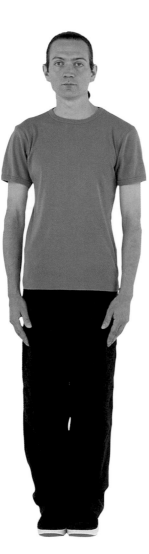

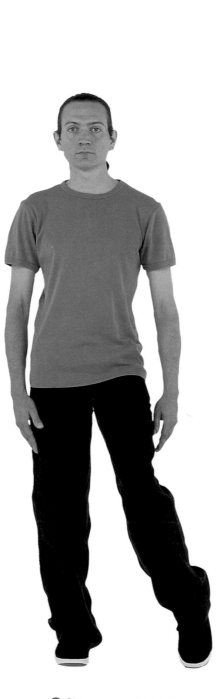

❸ Center your body weight.

❷ Sink your weight into your right leg and step out with your left foot to a shoulder's width.

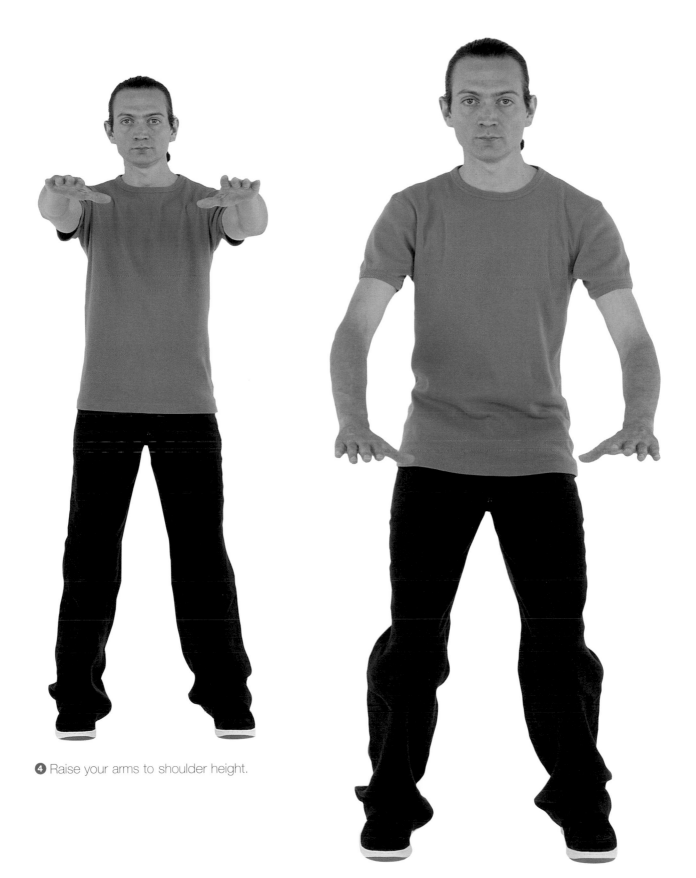

❹ Raise your arms to shoulder height.

❺ Bend your elbows and sit down into your posture.

2. raise hands

❶ The essence here is of opening and closing, both in the body and mind. Sink your weight onto your left leg and press gently back with your palms.

❷ Raise them up and outward (opening). Turn them inward and then bring your left hand in toward your right elbow (closing).

❸ At the same time, raise and place your right heel on the ground. Your body turns to a thirty-degree angle.

3. white crane spreads its wings

❶ Turn to the left and move into Hold the Ball.

❷ Turn your right foot around.

❸ Step back with your right foot and transfer your weight onto your right leg. As you do this, turn to the right and raise your right hand to head height.

❹ Turn to the left to face forward, bringing your left hand down and across. Relax and sink into your right leg.

4. brush knee and press

❶ Turn to the left and rotate your right forearm so that your palm is facing in.

❷ Bring the right palm down and raise the left hand. Turn to the right.

❸ As your right hand rises, step in with your left foot.

4 Step forward with your left foot and bend your right arm, bringing your left hand down to waist height.

5 Transfer your weight forward into a left-sided Bow Stance and press forward with your right palm.

5. block, parry, and punch

❶ Transfer your weight back and turn to the left.

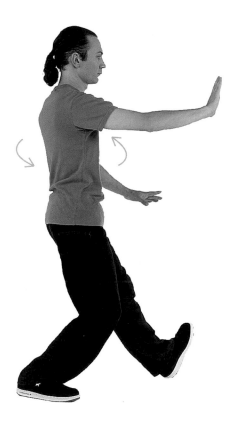

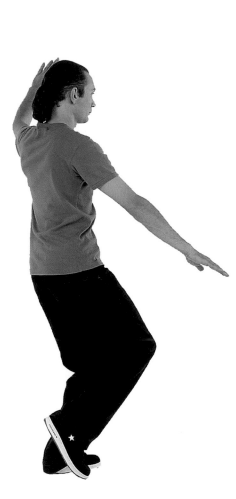

❷ As you bring your weight forward, raise your left hand up in an arc and circle down with your right hand. Step onto your left instep with your right foot.

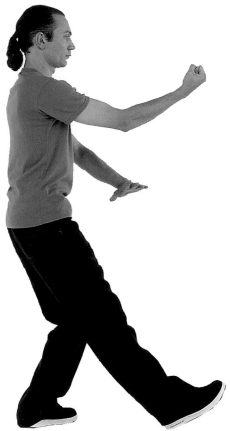

❸ Turn to the front and circle up, down, and out with your right fist (a backhand strike) as your left hand comes down. Place your right foot forward, heel down, in front of you, with the toe turned out to the right.

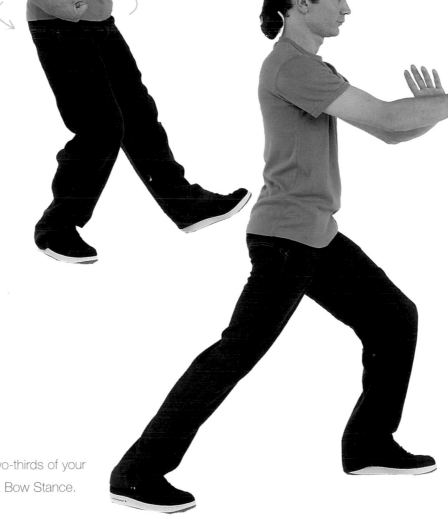

5 Turn to the left and step forward with the left foot, heel first. As this happens, the right fist comes to the right hip.

4 Turn to the right, pivoting and turning the right fist. As the left palm comes forward, transfer your weight onto your right leg and circle the right fist around.

6 Punch forward, transferring two-thirds of your weight onto the left leg to form a Bow Stance.

6. palm under elbow and push

❶ Open your fist and bring your left hand under your elbow.
Turn the left palm upward and bring it forward.

❷ Transfer your weight back, separating the palms.

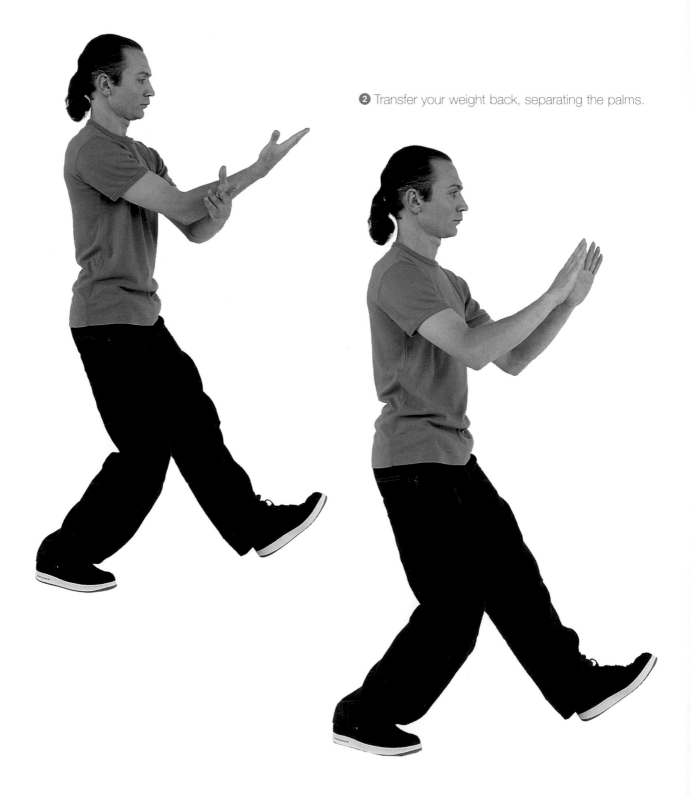

❸ Push down, as pictured below, and then forward and up to shoulder height.

❹ As you do this, two-thirds of your weight comes forward to form a Bow Stance.

7. cloud hands

The direction of this movement is the opposite to the Eight-Posture Form. The whole sequence is repeated two and a half times.

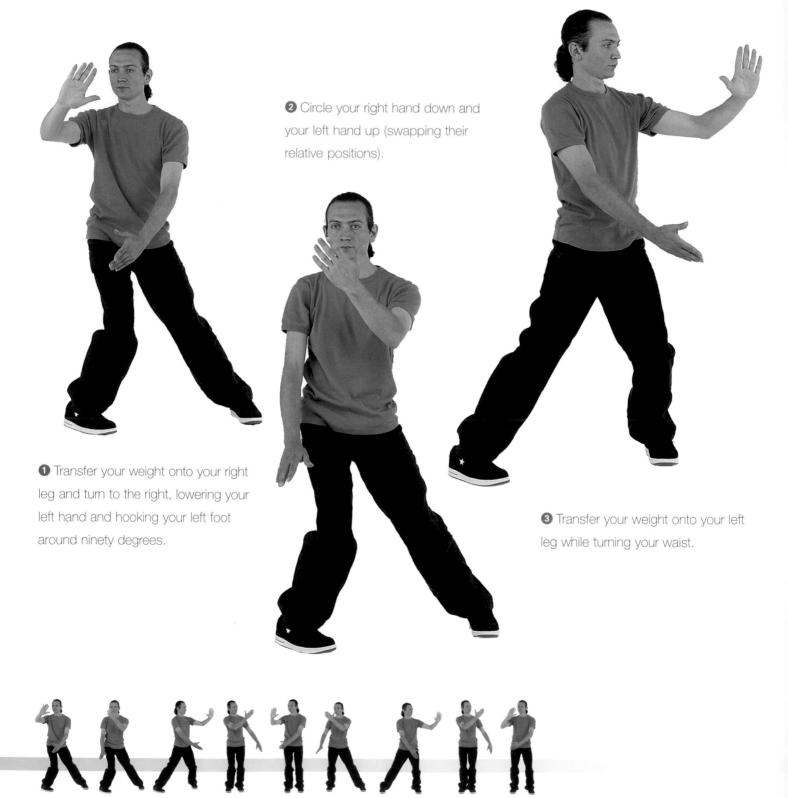

❷ Circle your right hand down and your left hand up (swapping their relative positions).

❶ Transfer your weight onto your right leg and turn to the right, lowering your left hand and hooking your left foot around ninety degrees.

❸ Transfer your weight onto your left leg while turning your waist.

1   2   3   4   5   6   7   8   9

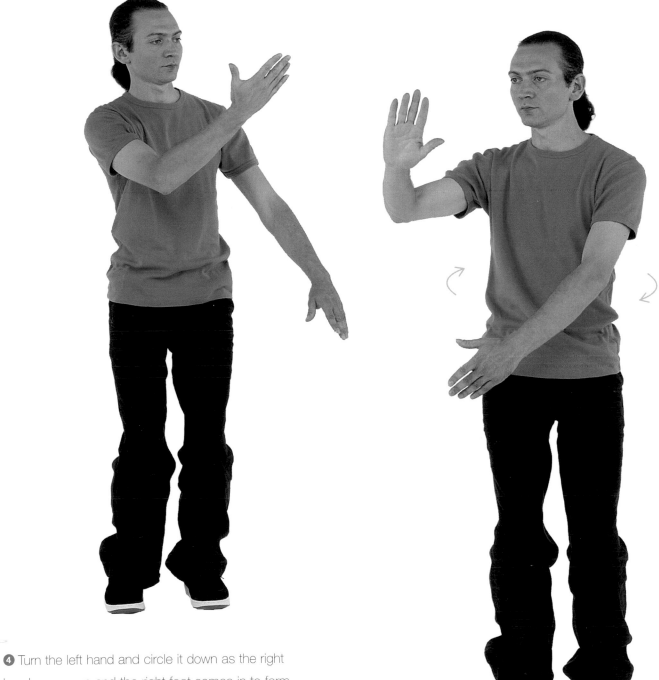

4 Turn the left hand and circle it down as the right hand comes up and the right foot comes in to form a parallel stance.

5 Turn to the right and turn the right palm out.

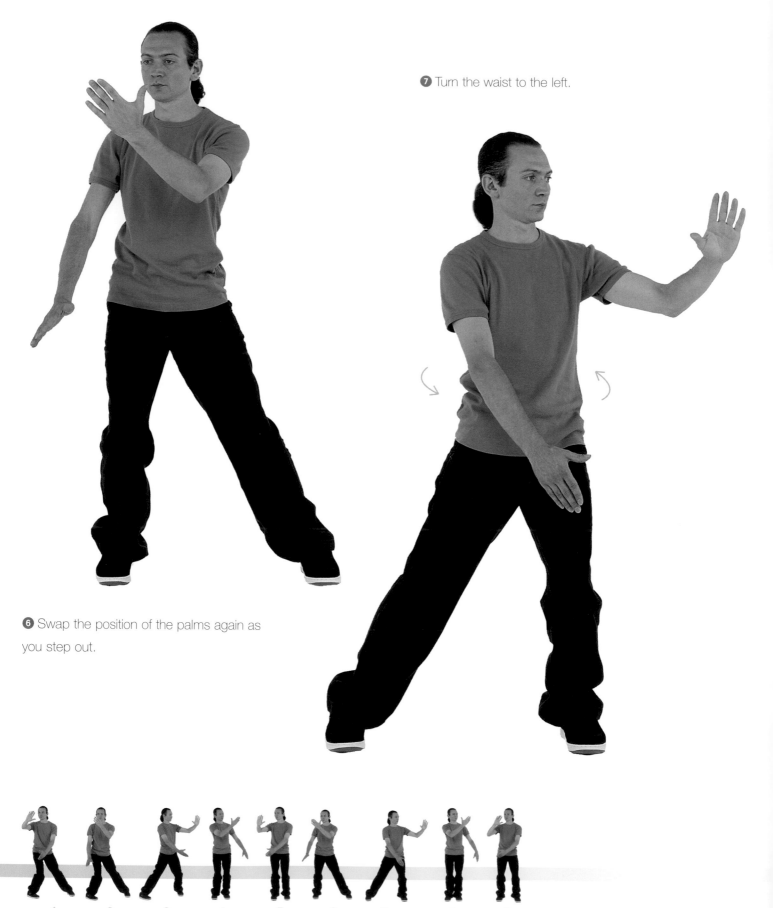

7 Turn the waist to the left.

6 Swap the position of the palms again as you step out.

❽ Again, swap the palms, step out with your right foot, and shift the weight again, looking at your right hand.

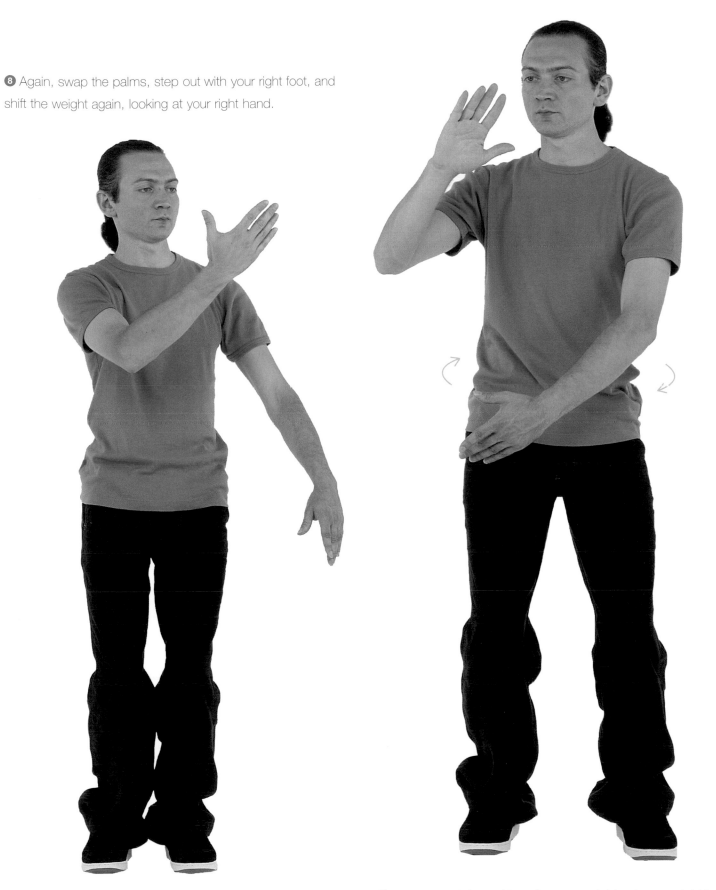

❾ Turn to the right and transfer your weight onto your right leg.

8. single whip

Here, Single Whip is reversed and is in the opposite direction to the Eight-Posture Form.

❶ From Cloud Hands, the weight is on the right leg and you are looking at your right hand.

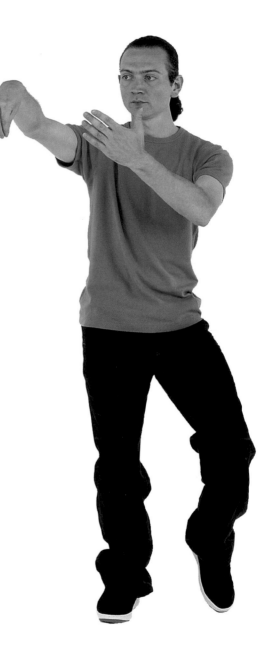

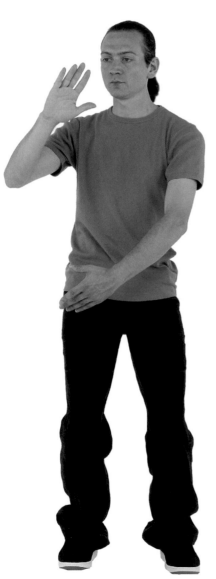

❷ Turn the right hand outward and raise the left hand. Step in with your left foot and form the Crane's Beak.

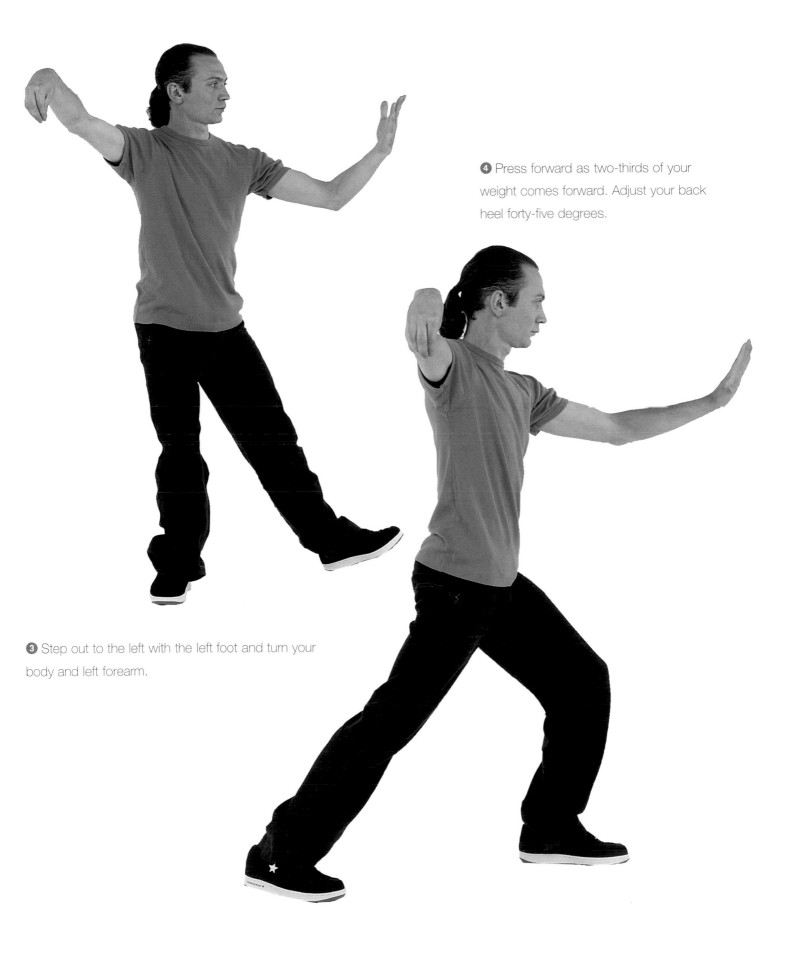

❹ Press forward as two-thirds of your weight comes forward. Adjust your back heel forty-five degrees.

❸ Step out to the left with the left foot and turn your body and left forearm.

9. strum the lute

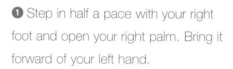

❶ Step in half a pace with your right foot and open your right palm. Bring it forward of your left hand.

❷ As you shift your weight back onto your right leg, push your left hand forward and past your right palm as you turn slightly to the right.

❸ Turn to the front and raise your left heel, placing it on the ground in front of you (a low kick).

10. repulse the monkey

This movement is a backward step and forward push while pulling in toward the body at the same time. The step backward moves in and out in an arc.

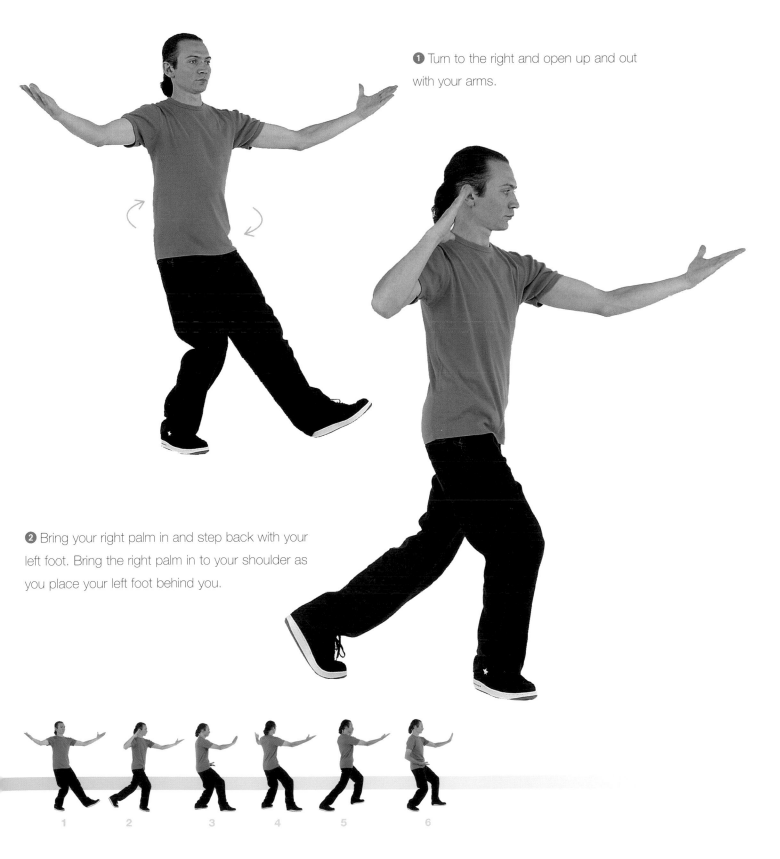

1 Turn to the right and open up and out with your arms.

2 Bring your right palm in and step back with your left foot. Bring the right palm in to your shoulder as you place your left foot behind you.

1   2   3   4   5   6

3 As you shift the weight back, push forward with the right hand past the left hand (which is coming in to the hip). You end up facing forward.

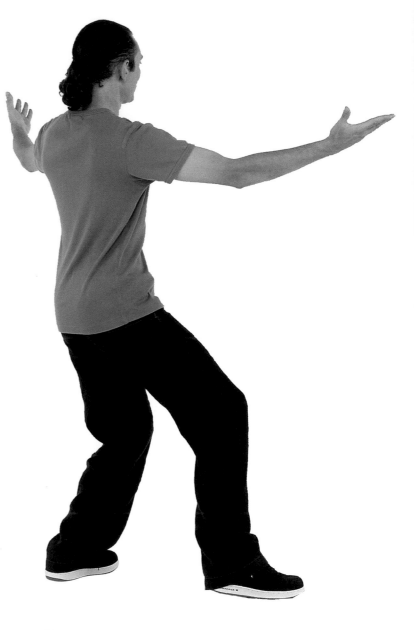

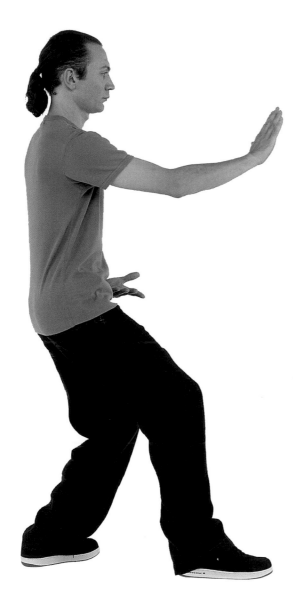

4 The move is repeated on the other side. Turn and open to the left, as shown.

1   2   3   4   5   6

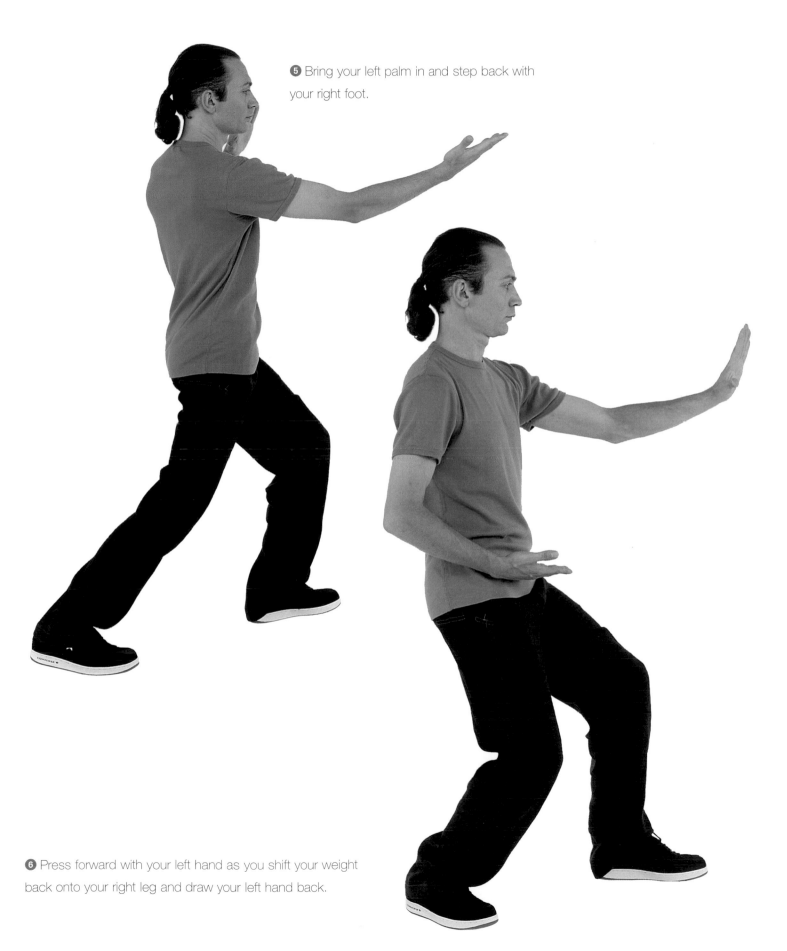

5 Bring your left palm in and step back with your right foot.

6 Press forward with your left hand as you shift your weight back onto your right leg and draw your left hand back.

11. snake creeps down golden rooster stands on one leg

This part of the form involves a low stance (Snake Creeps Down) and an upright, empty stance (Golden Rooster Stands on One Leg). Snake Creeps Down derives its name from the low stance, emulating the posture of a snake on the ground. Golden Rooster Stands on One Leg is very good for balance.

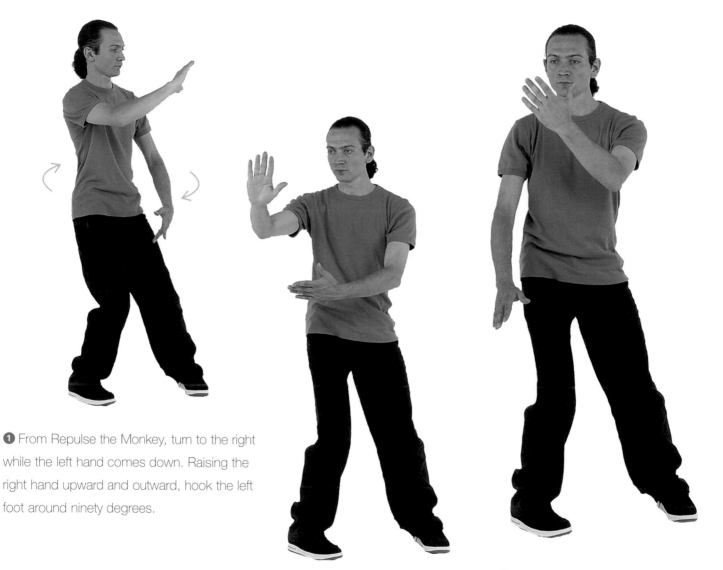

❶ From Repulse the Monkey, turn to the right while the left hand comes down. Raising the right hand upward and outward, hook the left foot around ninety degrees.

❷ Turn the right palm out.

❸ Swap the relative positions of the palms by circling the right hand down and the left hand up.

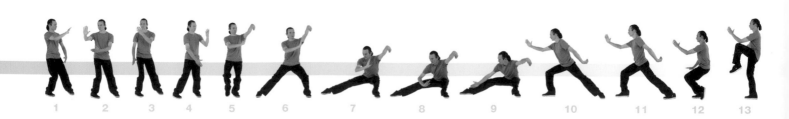

1   2   3   4   5   6   7   8   9   10   11   12   13

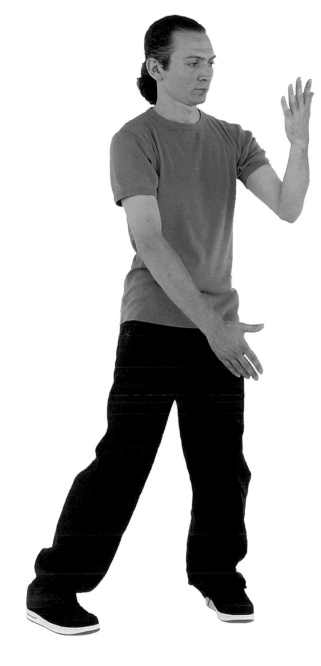

❹ Shift the weight onto the left leg and turn your waist.

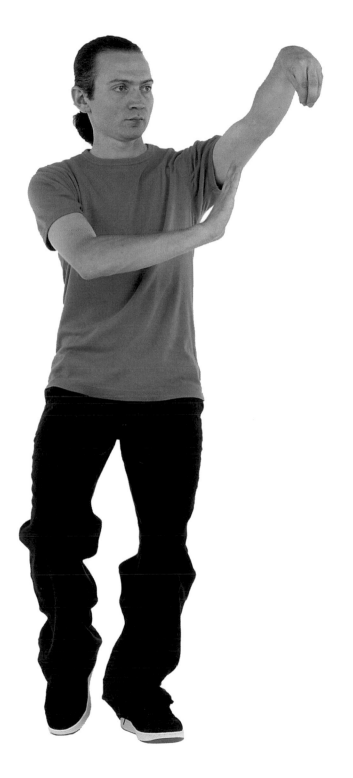

❺ Turn the left palm out and extend the arm. Raise your right hand and bring it in to beneath your left elbow.

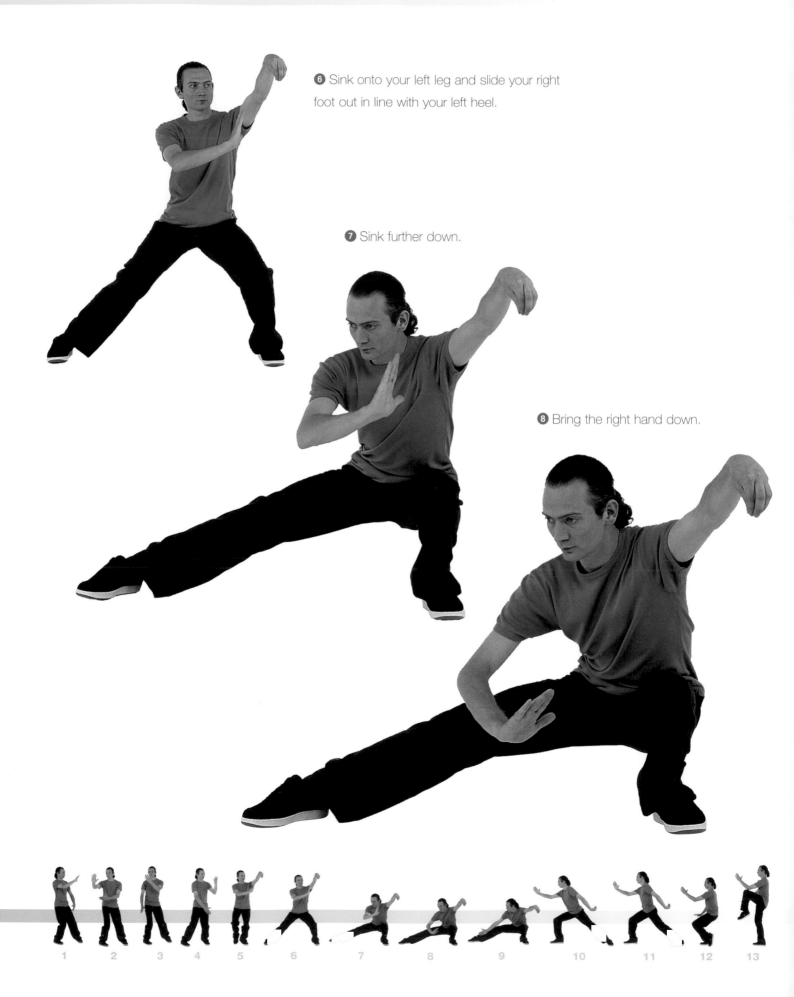

6 Sink onto your left leg and slide your right foot out in line with your left heel.

7 Sink further down.

8 Bring the right hand down.

1   2   3   4   5   6   7   8   9   10   11   12   13

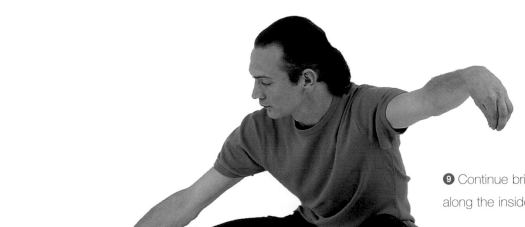

9 Continue bringing the right hand down along the inside of your right leg.

10 Turn to the right and turn your right foot ninety degrees. Bring two-thirds of your body weight onto your front leg to form a long Bow Stance. As this happens, bring the left "beak hand" down to behind your left thigh.

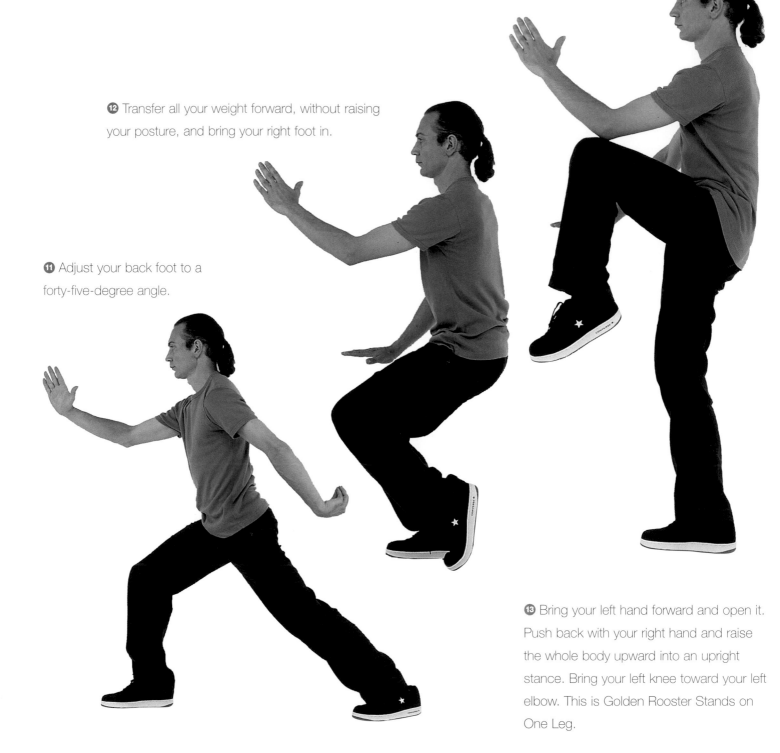

12 Transfer all your weight forward, without raising your posture, and bring your right foot in.

11 Adjust your back foot to a forty-five-degree angle.

13 Bring your left hand forward and open it. Push back with your right hand and raise the whole body upward into an upright stance. Bring your left knee toward your left elbow. This is Golden Rooster Stands on One Leg.

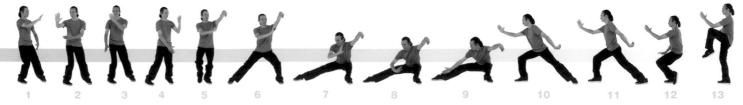

1   2   3   4   5   6   7   8   9   10   11   12   13

12. fair lady weaves the shuttles

This movement incorporates an upward and outward deflection with the right forearm (the forearm rotating as the waist turns), as if deflecting a blow from above. The left hand presses forward and you end up in a Bow Stance. The movement should consist of fluid turns.

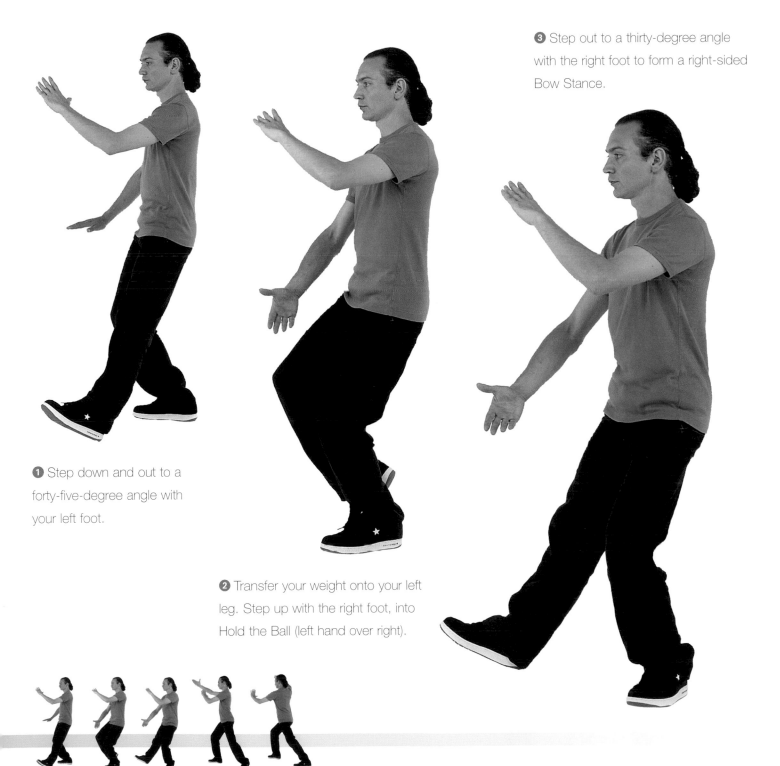

❸ Step out to a thirty-degree angle with the right foot to form a right-sided Bow Stance.

❶ Step down and out to a forty-five-degree angle with your left foot.

❷ Transfer your weight onto your left leg. Step up with the right foot, into Hold the Ball (left hand over right).

1   2   3   4   5

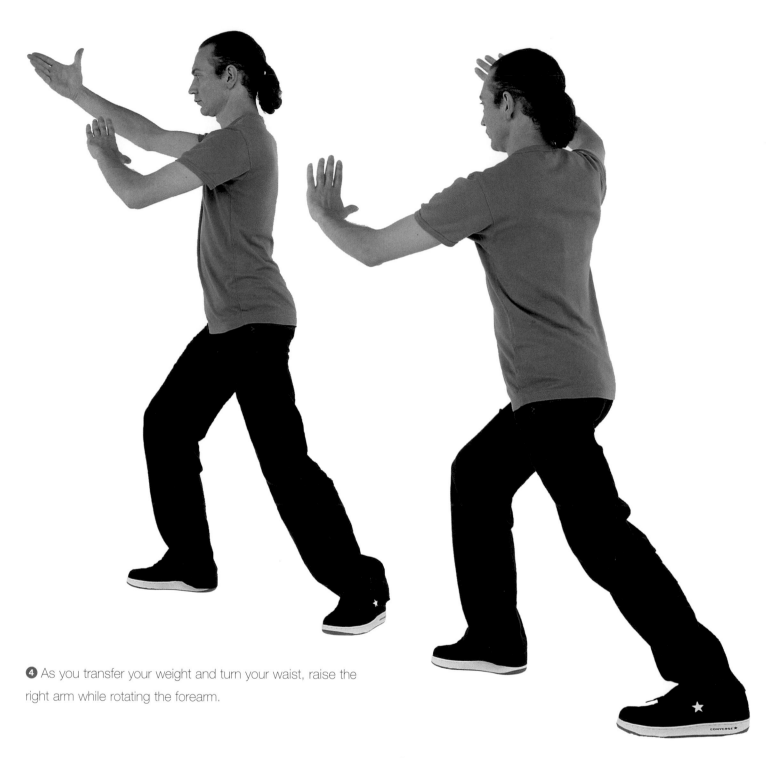

❹ As you transfer your weight and turn your waist, raise the right arm while rotating the forearm.

❺ Press forward with the left hand. The right hand arcs around to the side and to head height, with the palm facing out. Two-thirds of your body weight is forward.

1   2   3   4   5

13. the needle at the bottom of the sea

This movement is done in an empty stance and is characterized by a tilt of the posture forward as you point the left hand toward the ground. Mental energy should be focused on the floor, with particular emphasis on the downward push of the hands.

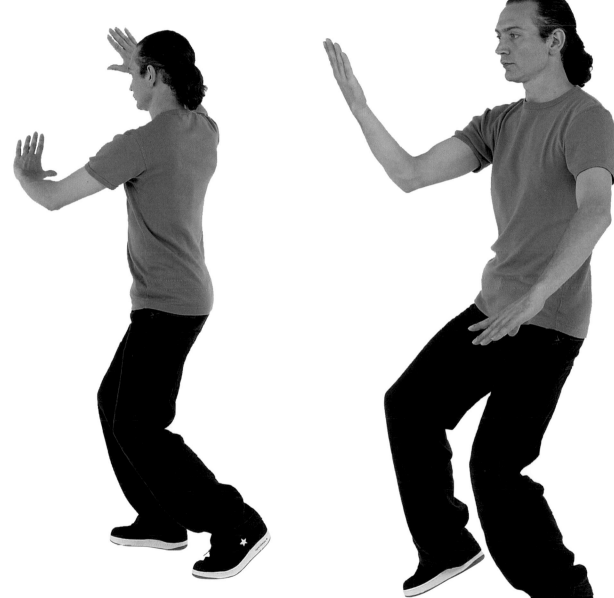

❶ Step up half a pace with the left foot, turning the foot out slightly, as shown.

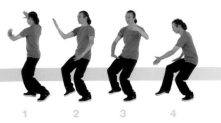

1   2   3   4

❷ As you transfer your weight back, turn your body and deflect to the left with your right arm.

❸ The left hand turns to the side with the movement of the body and arches upward.

❹ As you turn to the front, the right hand comes down and across to your right side while the right foot rises slightly and comes down. It is placed on the ground, with the toe down and the heel raised. The left hand strikes forward and downward simultaneously with the rest of the movement.

1   2   3   4

14. fan penetrates the back

Here there is a subtle step in as your right fingers connect with your left wrist. The stance at the end is Bow Stance. The energy here is one of separation and splitting as the right hand grabs an arm and the left hand presses forward. The hands in this position are meant to emulate the shape of a Chinese fan.

1 Turning slightly to the left, raise the right and left hands in front of the forehead, stepping in with the left foot.

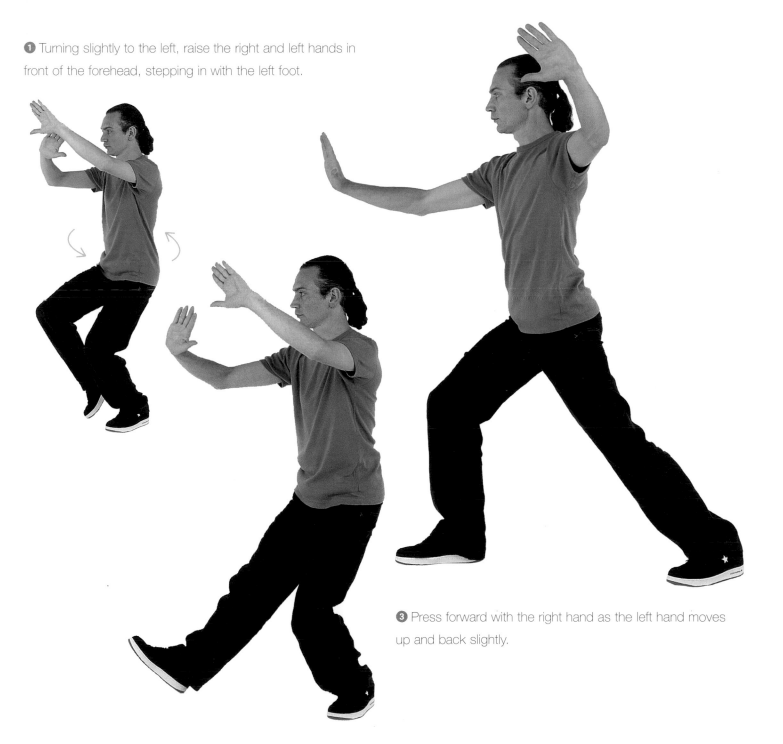

3 Press forward with the right hand as the left hand moves up and back slightly.

2 Step forward to form a right-sided Bow Stance.

15. cross arm posture

❶ Center your body weight and turn to the left, hooking your right foot around ninety degrees to the left.

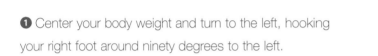

❷ Turn your left foot around ninety degrees to the right. Continue to smoothly transfer two-thirds of your weight onto the left leg to form a Bow Stance and open the arms slightly outward.

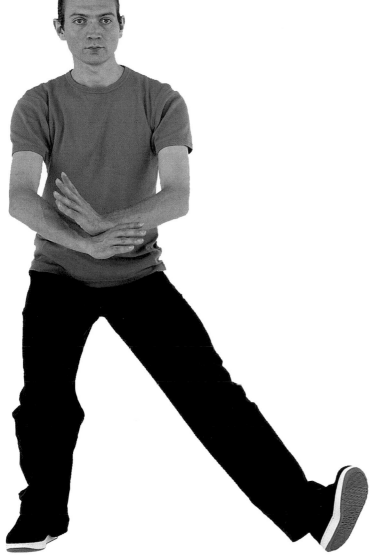

3 Transfer your weight onto your right leg and raise the left toes, circling the hands down and in.

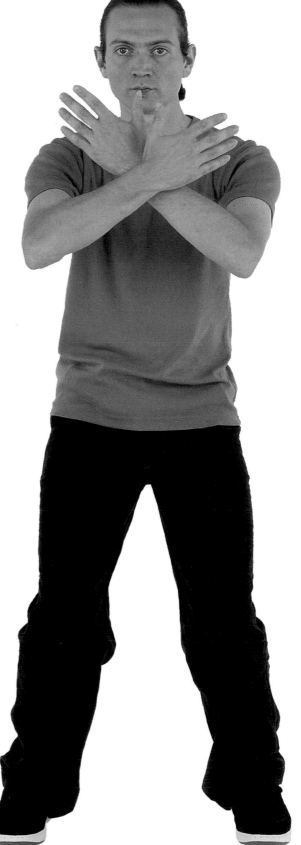

4 Step in with the left foot to form a shoulder-width stance as you cross your hands in front of you, right hand on the outside.

16. close

The energy built up throughout the exercises performed can be held and enjoyed at the beginning of this pose. The hands are then lowered, with the palms pressing down into the ground, signifying the slow release of the stored energy that has been built up.

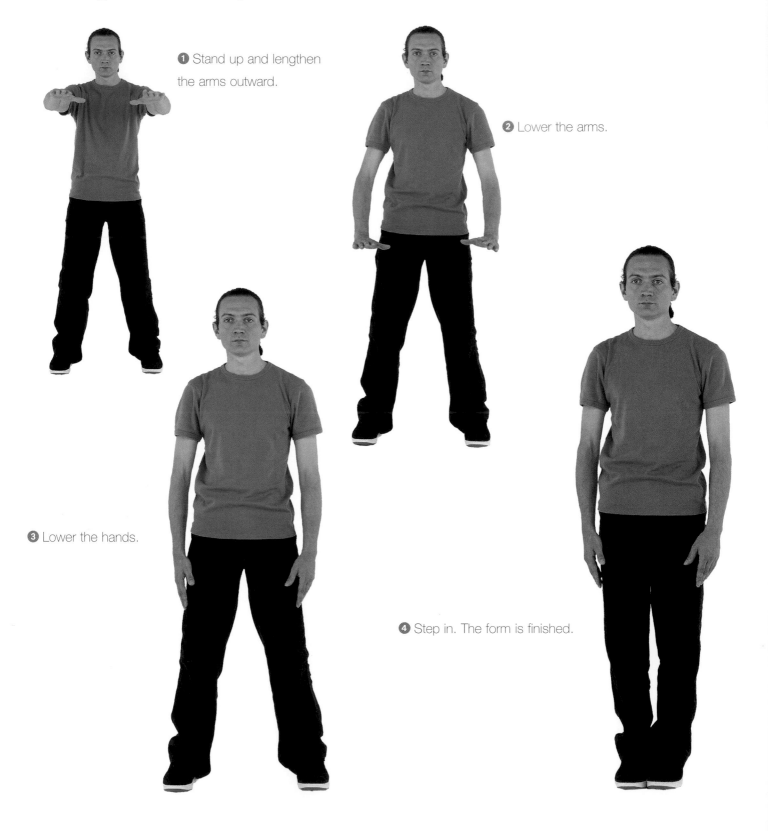

1 Stand up and lengthen the arms outward.

2 Lower the arms.

3 Lower the hands.

4 Step in. The form is finished.

In cultivating your mind, know how to be gentle and kind.
In speaking, know how to keep your words.
In governing, know how to maintain order.
In transacting business, know how to choose the right moment.

Tao Te Ching

partner work

working with a partner

Practicing tai chi with a friend is enormously helpful and may well help you to progress quickly. Simply going through your movements together is motivating, and talking about the moves is helpful in clarifying some of the points you are learning. There are also ways of working together that include posture testing and giving feedback on posture and movement.

Partner work allows you to feel and understand how tai chi principles such as listening, yielding, and applying force really work. Such exercises add another dimension to your practice and will help you to experience how your body and mind can work as a whole, in response to an incoming force. By relaxing, "sinking," yielding, or turning the waist an incoming force can be absorbed, redirected, or neutralized without you losing your own root and balance. This sense of retaining your own equilibrium in the face of an incoming force is fundamental to tai chi.

posture checking

Poor posture is a common problem that tai chi undoubtedly helps. Leaning forward, as in ❶, or back, as in ❷ and ❹, will hinder your movement, make it harder to turn easily on the central axis of your body, and may lead to excessive strain being placed on the lumbar or thoracic vertebrae. Often we are not even aware our posture is poor, so having a friend check for you is really important (❸ and ❺). This will help you reeducate your body and lead to increased awareness of some of the basic points of tai chi practice.

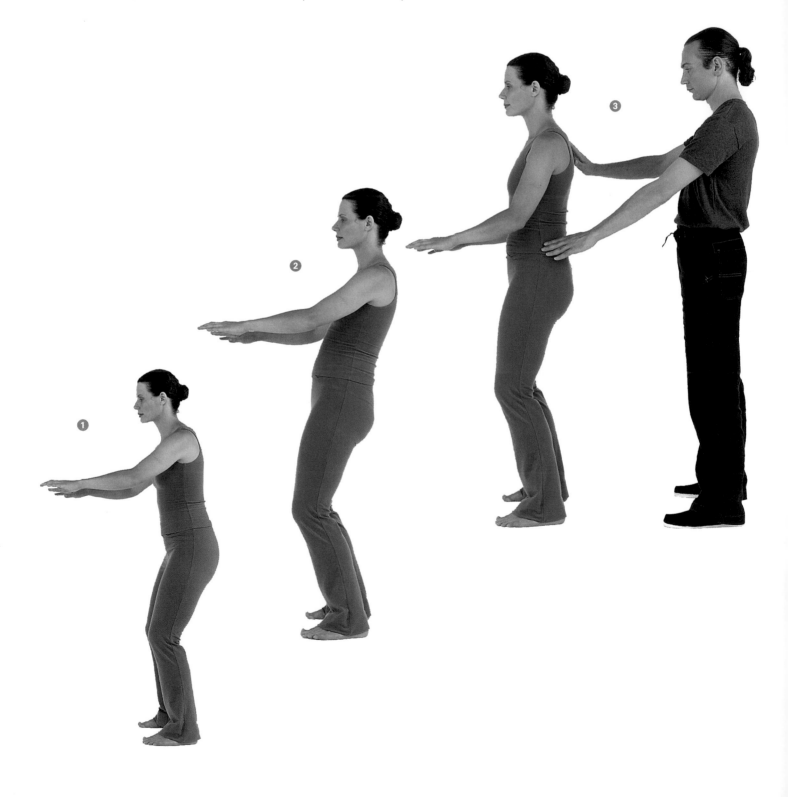

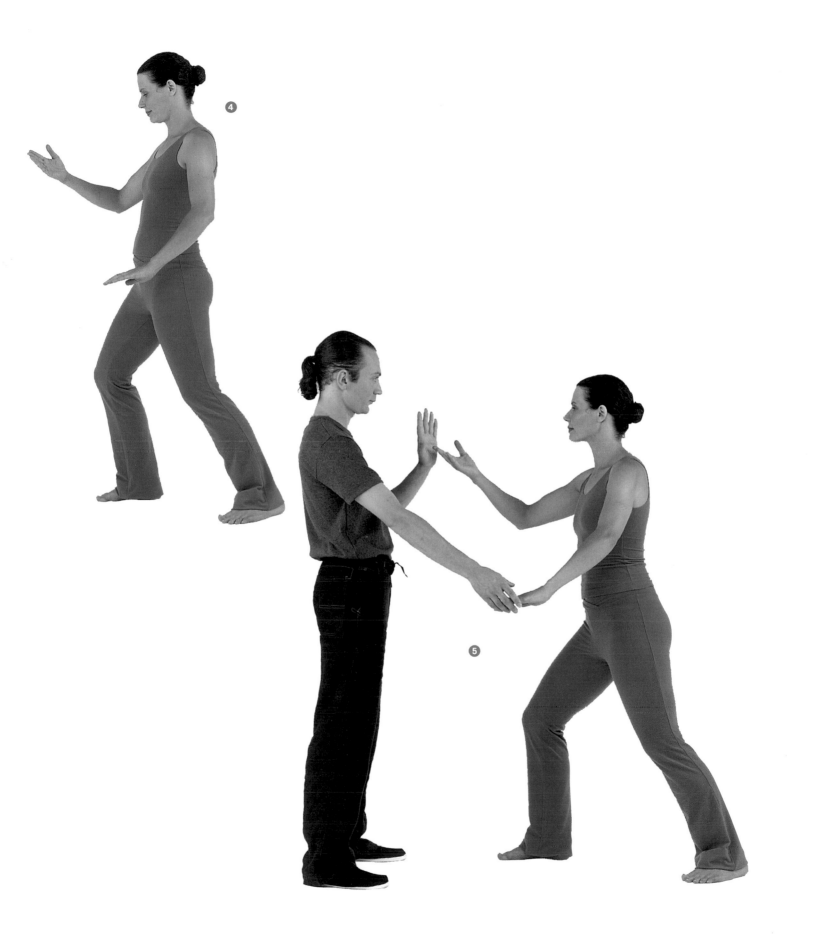

posture testing

Once you have gained a good grounding in your tai chi stances, you may wish to test their natural strength by getting a friend to steadily push into your arm as you hold one of the stances. This is a good way of establishing whether your stance is strong and aligned correctly, and also good for developing an awareness of Peng (Ward Off Energy). In an experienced practitioner, the stance should be very strong but relaxed and the body should have a natural springiness and resistance (Peng). This is essentially achieved by relaxing and sinking, but maintaining your shape (this could be compared to squeezing a tennis ball—when force is applied, the ball compresses and then springs back into shape because of its natural strength).

   In the early stages, the alignment of the body is of prime importance. If, for example, the back knee in Bow Stance is allowed to collapse inward, the stance will have no strength and no structure. Without structure, there is no form. Below, you can see a tai chi practitioner pressing into the arm of his partner to test the alignment of her stance. The press should be felt in the back foot. As the pressure of the press is increased, the structure will either hold its own or collapse—giving you the opportunity to improve the stance by adjusting the posture or develop Peng.

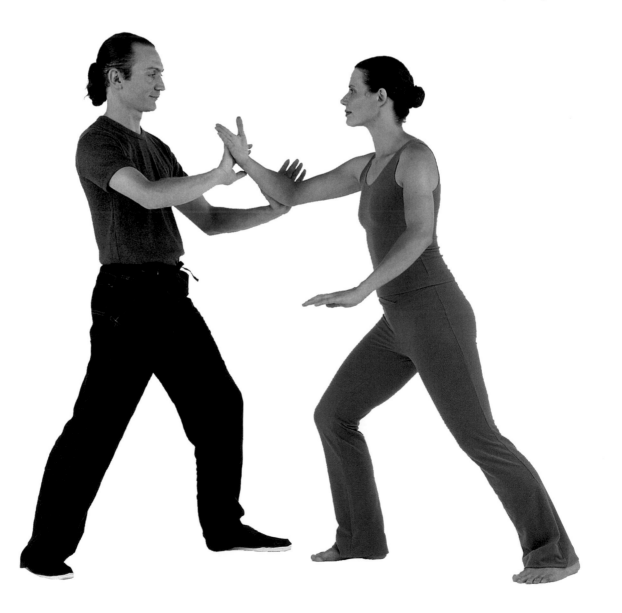

push hands exercises

These Push Hands exercises are great for developing the qualities learned in your form when working with a partner. They also serve as a springboard to understanding how to yield, adhere (stick), and issue (fa jin) energy. Push Hands can help you become more aware of your posture when redirecting an incoming force (push). You also learn how to listen to what is going on between you so you can anticipate and respond to the incoming push of your partner.

At an advanced level, Push Hands forms the basis of martial skill while adding another dimension to your practice.

❶ The basic movement is circular, using Parting the Wild Horse's Mane as a basis. The feet do not move but the weight shifts forward and back. The waist should be allowed to turn freely, using the spine as an axis.

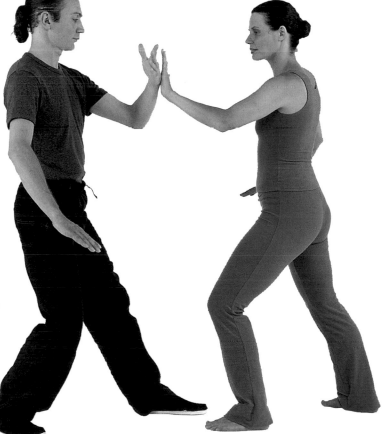

❷ As one person pushes forward, the other begins to yield, sitting back slightly.

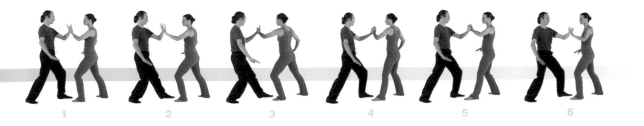

1   2   3   4   5   6

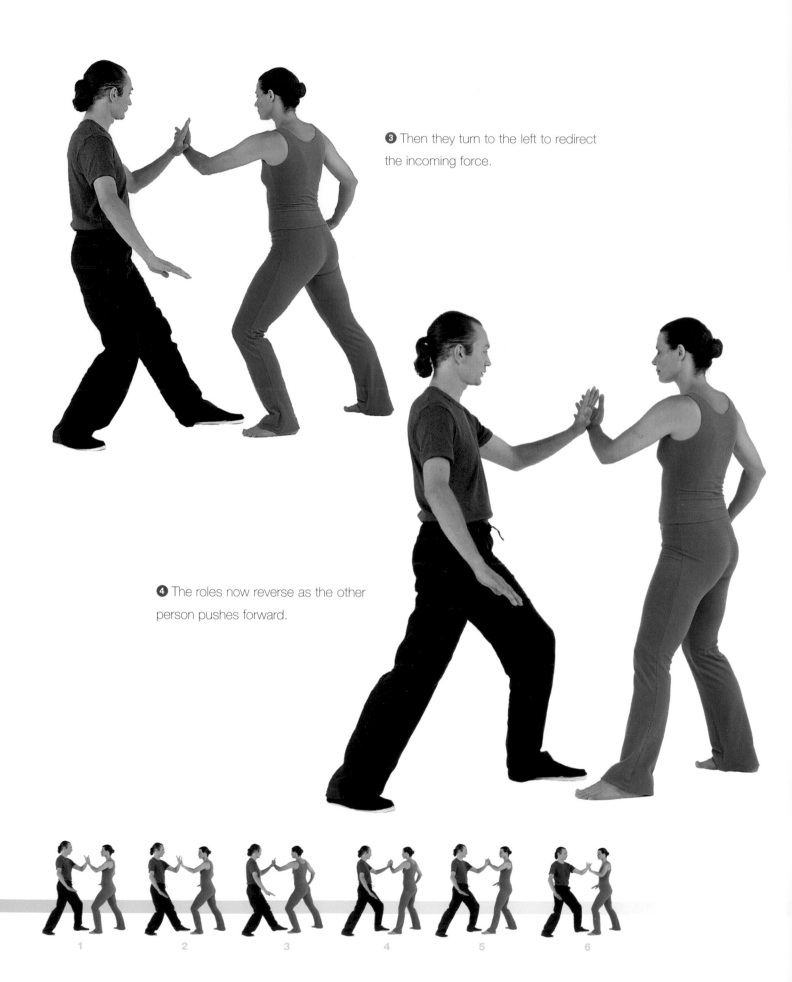

3 Then they turn to the left to redirect the incoming force.

4 The roles now reverse as the other person pushes forward.

1   2   3   4   5   6

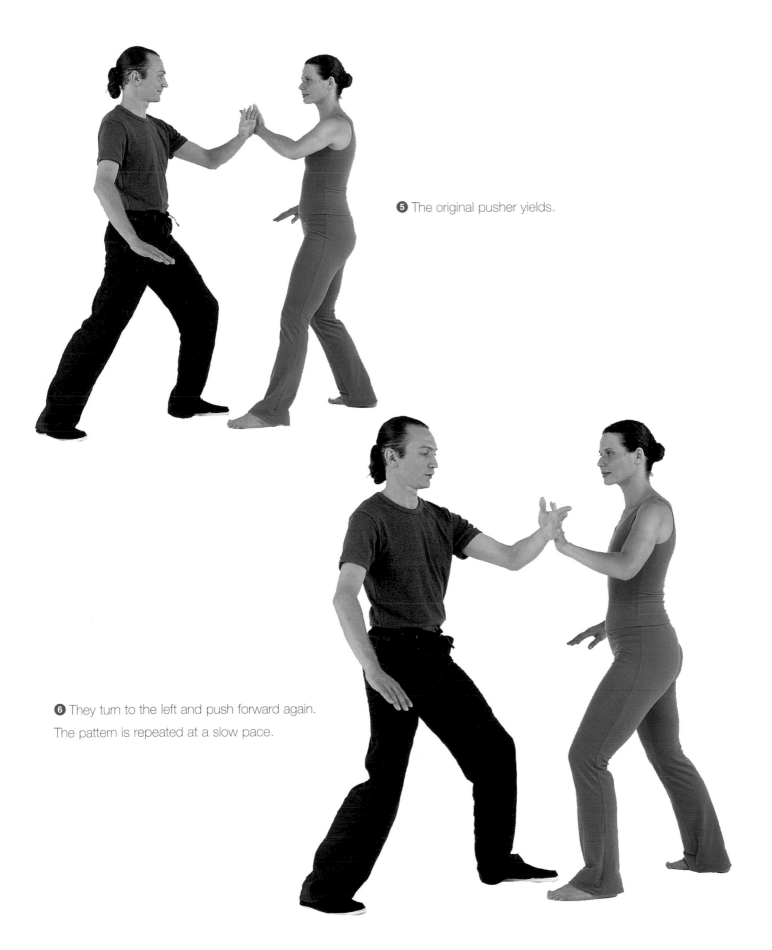

5 The original pusher yields.

6 They turn to the left and push forward again.
The pattern is repeated at a slow pace.

tai chi self-defense moves

Tai chi was originally used as a martial art and is still revered as such. Essentially defensive but with offensive countermoves, tai chi traditionally takes longer to master as a martial art than other fighting systems, although all movements in tai chi have covert martial applications within them. Learning tai chi as a martial art can help improve confidence, but you should be wary—it takes many years of practice before you can effectively employ tai chi as a way of protecting yourself.

The following photos and instructions will help you understand how tai chi can work on an obvious level. The more subtle aspects of tai chi boxing are reliant on the harnessing and development of the Eight Energies and techniques learned in Push Hands.

1. parting the wild horse's mane

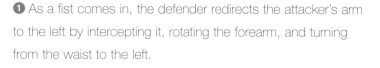

❶ As a fist comes in, the defender redirects the attacker's arm to the left by intercepting it, rotating the forearm, and turning from the waist to the left.

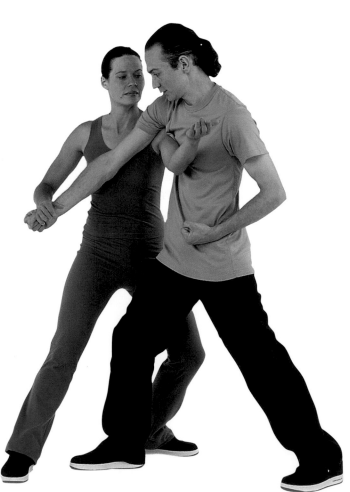

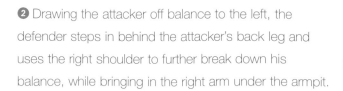

❷ Drawing the attacker off balance to the left, the defender steps in behind the attacker's back leg and uses the right shoulder to further break down his balance, while bringing in the right arm under the armpit.

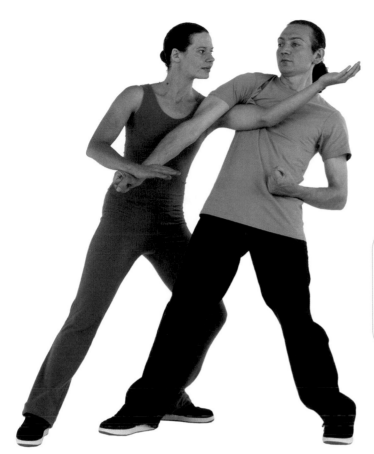

3 The defender then turns his or her body to throw the attacker further off balance.

> "Good warriors do not arm, good fighters don't get mad."
>
> *Tao Te Ching*, Verse 68, "Good Warriors"

2. white crane spreads its wings

1 The left arm is used to deflect the first punch with a turn to the left and rotation of the left forearm. The second punch is deflected in a similar manner downward. This splits and separates the incoming force, leaving the attacker vulnerable to a kick.

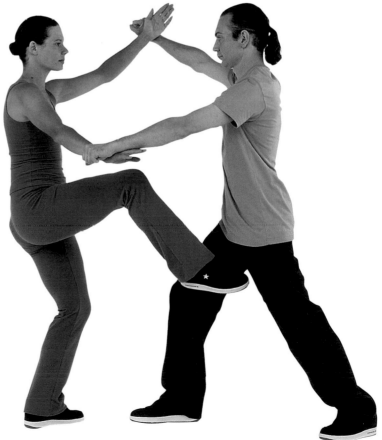

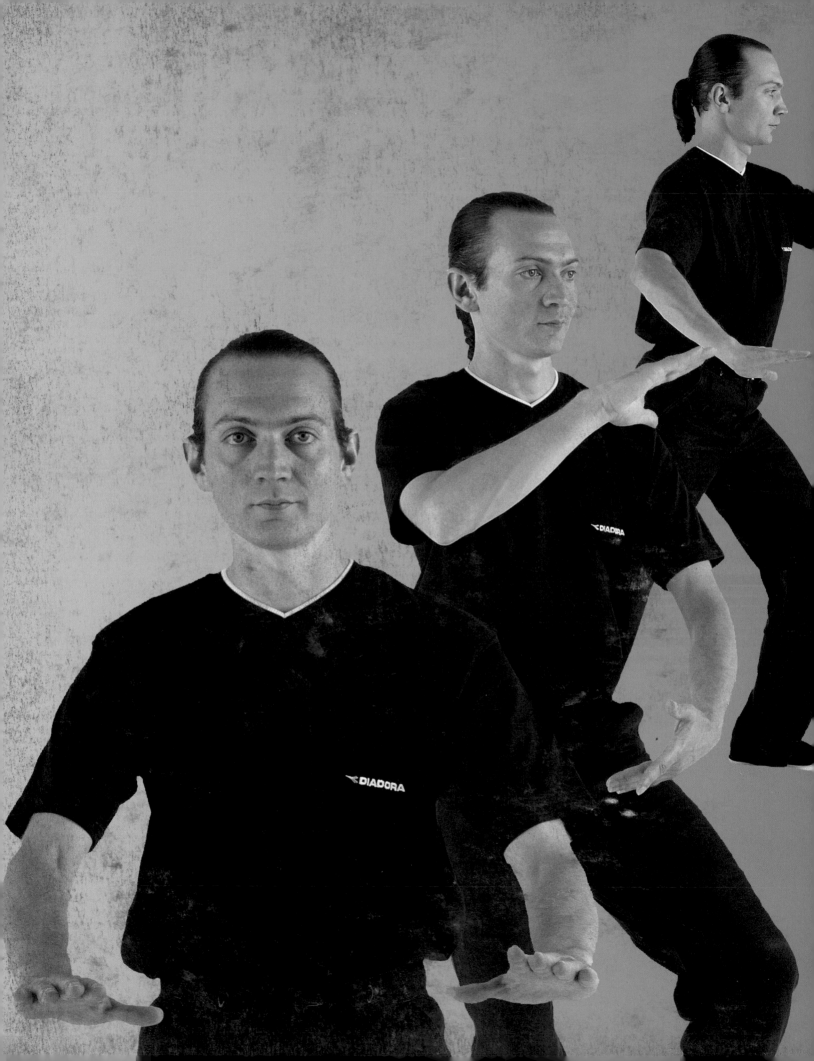

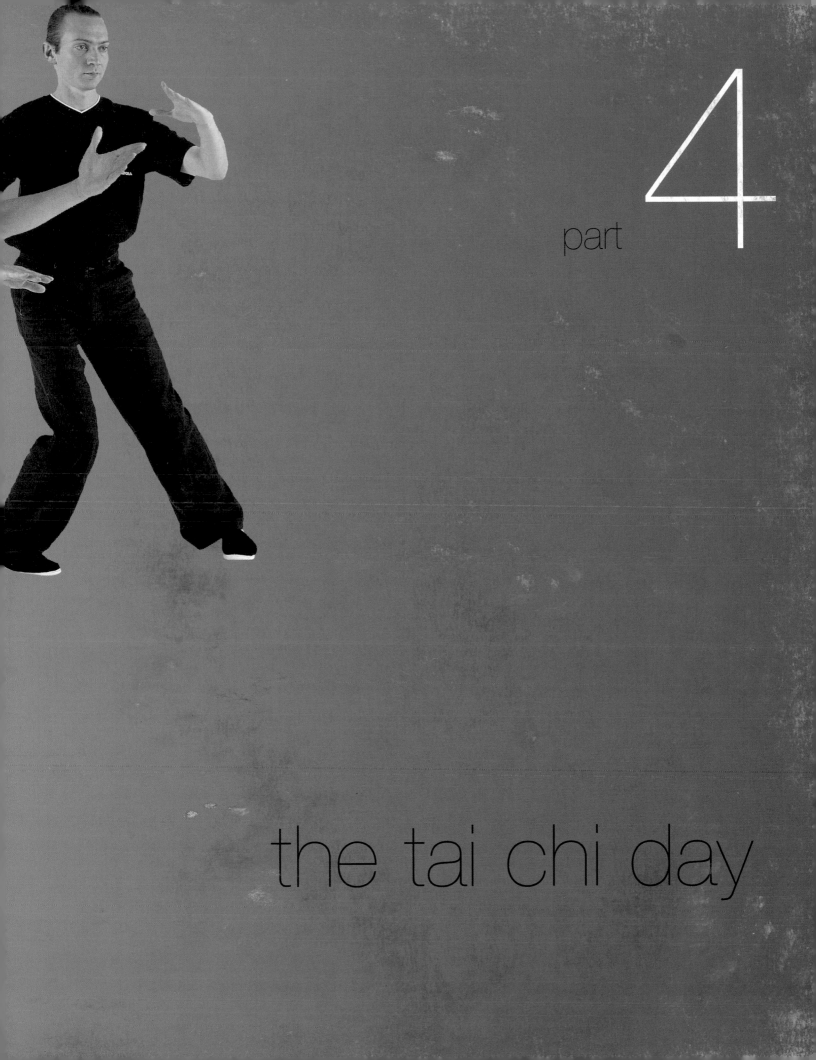

the tai chi day

tai chi for everyday life

tai chi for everyday life

All the exercises in this book can be followed as they are laid out, section by section. You may, however, wish to devise short routines for different times, especially if you have only a small amount of practice time available to you. These programs are suggestions to get you started, but you may find the exercises I have chosen particularly effective for specific times of the day. You can, of course, devise your own program based on what you have time for and your personal needs. The seated exercises that follow on the next page are especially suited for the elderly.

morning

It is important to get your energy moving in the morning in a natural way, rather than just relying on a stimulant such as caffeine. Because tai chi and Chi Kung rely on natural ways to improve your energy levels, you should feel the benefits both in body and mind.

afternoon

If your energy is low in the afternoon, some simple stretches will help release blocked energy. The mirror-image postures (pages 67–77) will enhance the circulation of your blood and chi.

evening

The evening session may well be when you need tai chi the most. Your shoulders, wrists, and ankles will benefit from some attention and practicing what you have learned form the Eight- and Sixteen-Posture Forms will help you feel more relaxed.

seated tai chi exercises

These are essentially the same as the tai chi upper-body movements.

open tai chi (page 63)

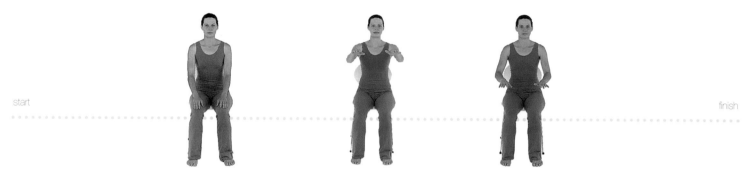

start   finish

white crane spreads its wings (page 66)

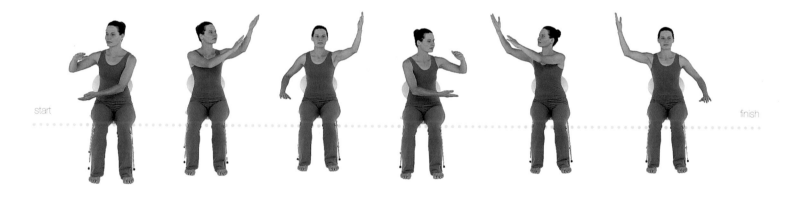

start   finish

cloud hands (page 72)

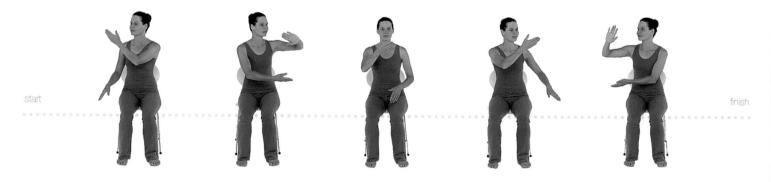

start   finish

the tai chi day

morning routine

1 Neck stretches. After waking up, you may find that your neck needs some attention, so the neck exercises are particularly important. The neck is a crucial area, as many of the meridians pass through it, as well as the main arteries of the body. This exercise will strengthen the energy in the bladder meridian. 2 minutes.

2 Open tai chi (simple upper-body movements, as on page 63). This will help get the energy flowing to your fingertips and release any stiffness from your shoulders and arms. It will also help with backaches and help energize your system. 2 minutes.

3 Tai chi form. It is a good idea to go through as many of the form movements as you have learned, or any of the mirror-image postures and upper-body movements. This will benefit your whole system and leave you feeling refreshed. 4 minutes.

4 Holding the Tan Tien (page 57). This exercise will help you feel calm and centered, ready for your day. 4 minutes.

Total: 12 minutes

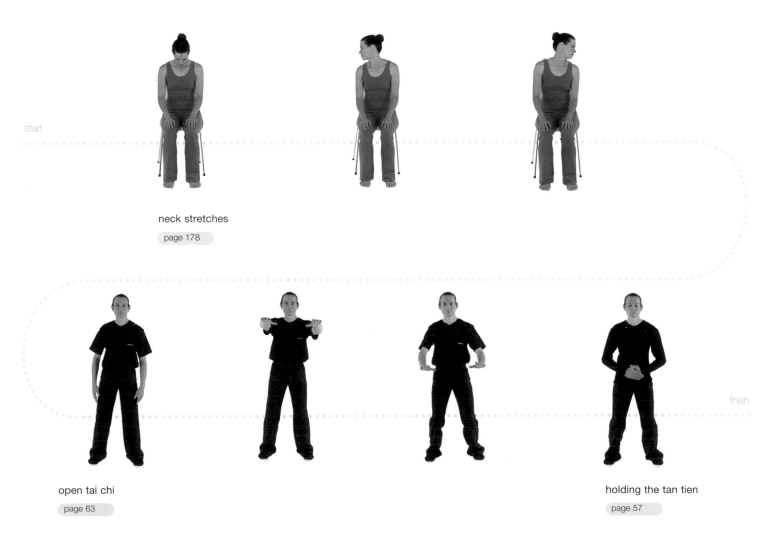

start

neck stretches
page 178

open tai chi
page 63

holding the tan tien
page 57

finish

afternoon routine

1 Stretching Upward and Forward is especially effective if you have been sitting at work or driving a lot, as they will release stress from your back and shoulders. 2 minutes.

2 Self-massage. These will simultaneously relieve fatigue and make you feel rebalanced. 4 minutes.

3 Mirror-image postures. As well as teaching you the skills of coordination and balance, these exercises will also help to strengthen the muscles in your legs and lower back. 5 minutes.

Total: 11 minutes

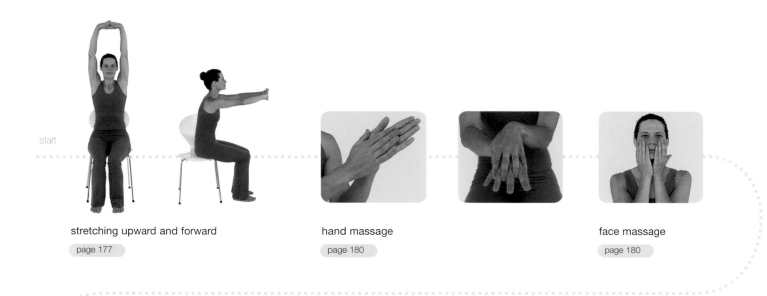

start

stretching upward and forward
page 177

hand massage
page 180

face massage
page 180

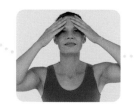 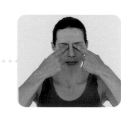 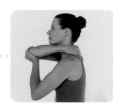 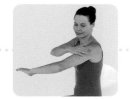 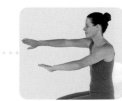

finish

shoulder and arm massage
page 181

mirror image, parting the wild horse's mane (pages 86–89)

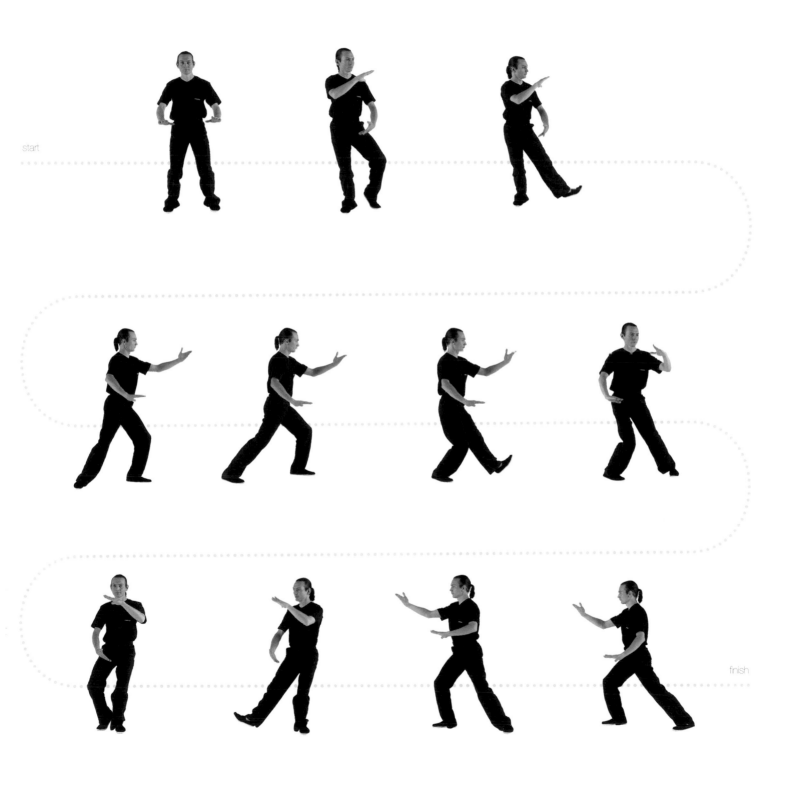

start

finish

asana
evening routine

1 Shoulder Circles (page 58). This will help free up any tension in your shoulders. 2 minutes.

2 Wrist and Ankle Rotations (page 59). If you have been using a keyboard at work, it is a good idea to work on your wrists to help release any stiffness. 2 minutes.

2 Tai chi form. 8 minutes.

4 Holding the Ball Chi Kung (page 60). This exercise is very good for your peace of mind, helping you feel calm before getting a good night's sleep. 4 minutes.

Total: 16 minutes

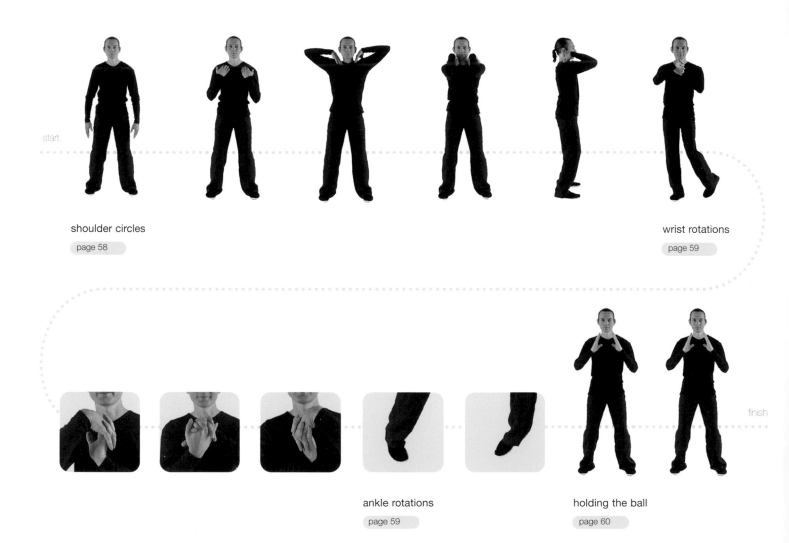

start

shoulder circles

page 58

wrist rotations

page 59

ankle rotations

page 59

holding the ball

page 60

finish

shoulder circles

❶ Begin with your fingers on your collarbone.

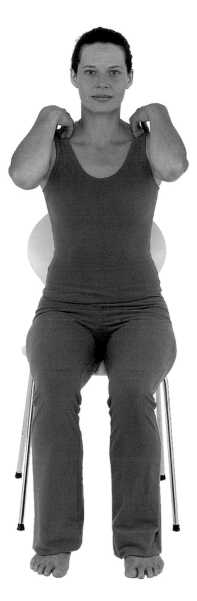

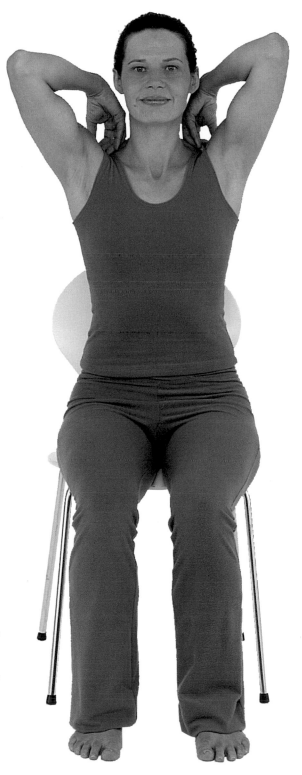

❷ Bring your elbows down, slightly back, and up, as if drawing a circle with your elbows. Repeat in the opposite direction.

self-massage

❶ Begin by rubbing your palms together and between your fingers.

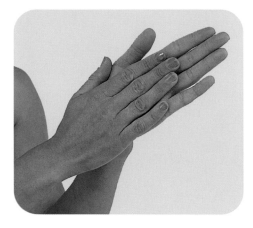 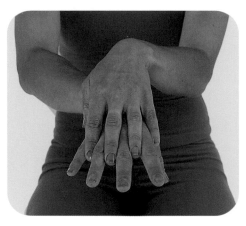

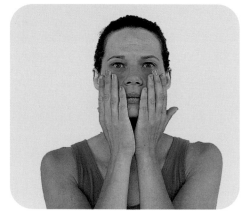 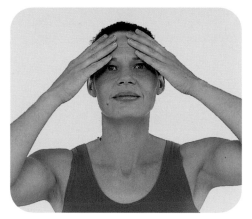 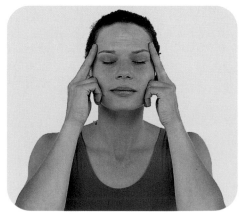

❷ From the center of your forehead, massage outward with your fingers to activate the acupressure points on the forehead.

❸ Massage your temples (this is good for migraines).

4 Press gently into the accupressure point in the bridge of the nose three times.

5 Press gently into the accupressure point at the base of the nostril three times.

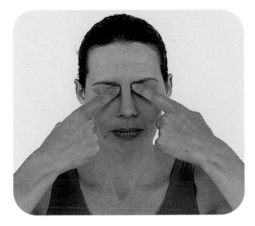

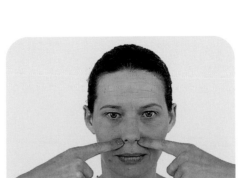

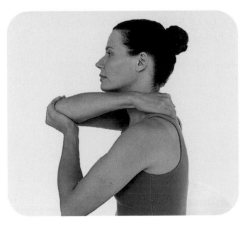

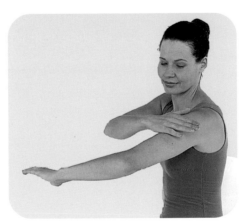

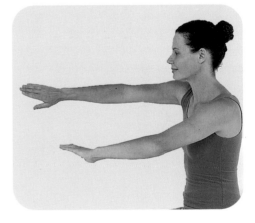

6 Grip the shoulder muscles with the fingers and the heel of the hand and work into any tender or stiff areas, working down the shoulder.

7 Hold your left arm straight out in front of you at shoulder height. Stroke gently your right palm down the length of your left arm, pressing down firmly.

8 Repeat for the other side.

guided meditation

The process of learning tai chi can be enhanced by visualization, a technique now used in many different fields. Since tai chi is about mind as well as body, this guided meditation can serve as a way of reinforcing your learning.

Meditation can be adapted to suit your needs once you are familiar with the formula. The main emphasis is to create a good energy around you and to gradually build up a picture of yourself doing your form. This will strengthen your mental familiarization with the sequence, as well as improve your powers of concentration. Don't expect too much too soon. Try to gradually increase your progress, movement by movement, until you can complete the sequence in your mind. To begin, make sure you will remain undisturbed for at least twenty minutes. Find a comfortable place to sit. It is best to do this meditation sitting, rather than lying down, as this encourages you to remain awake. Sit on the edge of your seat, with your feet flat on the ground and your back straight but relaxed. Your hands should be placed inward, just below your belly button.

Sit peacefully and focus your attention on your posture and your breathing. Just be aware of the natural rhythm of your breath and the area just below your navel (the Tan Tien). Sit quietly, relaxing and being aware of your Tan Tien.

Now imagine a special place, a place of special significance to you. Think of somewhere you would want to practice your tai chi. This could be a real or an imaginary place, inside or outside. Choose a peaceful place where there is no disturbance except for perhaps a gentle breeze or a distant sound of birdsong or running water. Beautiful trees may surround this place, or rich meadow grass, or it may simply be a quiet room. This is a safe place for you and also a place of positive experience and ease.

Try to imagine this place with as many senses as possible. What does it look like? What colors surround you? What textures do you see? What fragrances can you smell? What sounds can you hear? What atmosphere can you sense? This special place should feel safe and secure. It should be a magical place that can help you reach your potential and develop your awareness. The more senses you involve, the more successful your meditation will be.

Now see yourself standing in this place, peaceful and alert, ready for your tai chi form. See yourself moving into the opening movement of the form, slowly sinking your weight onto your right leg, maintaining a good posture, stepping out and centering your body weight, and raising your palms to shoulder level. Keep visualizing yourself in this manner, completing each movement with as much detail as you can muster—imagining, sensing, and feeling the movements imbued with the qualities you desire. Do this for as many movements of your form as you can. Don't worry if you can only visualize two or three of the movements. This will increase with time and practice. When you have reached the end of this visualization, slowly bring yourself back to the sensations in your body and the sounds in the room. Slowly open your eyes, bringing awareness back into the present. You should feel relaxed, calm, and energized.

This is a meditative exercise for centering and focusing the mind. Begin with your palms on your lower abdomen, just below your navel. Close your eyes, relax, and focus your attention on the sensations in your hands and in the area of your body beneath your hands. Try to keep your mind gently focused. If your mind wanders, gently bring it back to the exercise. Do this for about four minutes and then gently bring your awareness back into the room and open your eyes. You should feel relaxed and calm.

Between heaven and earth, there seems to be a bellows.
It is empty, it is empty, and yet it is inexhaustible.
No amount of words can fathom it.
Better look for it within you.

Tao Te Ching

practicing tai chi

how much? how often?
the art of discipline

Practicing is the only way to feel the benefits. It is a simple rule but one that seems to elude us, especially when we want to feel the benefits, reap the rewards, and when we are good at being lazy, procrastinating, and giving way to excuses. Most people usually practice "tomorrow" and the dropout rate in most tai chi classes is as high as in any other class whether it be aerobics, meditation, or salsa dancing.

How much you practice is entirely up to you, but ten minutes a day is a start. You get out what you put in (actually, I would say you get out much more than you put in). Traditionally, there was no limit to practice; in fact, to many tai chi masters, practicing is a way of life and may take up most of the day. However much you practice, be appreciative of the effort you have put in, the willingness you have to practice, and the desire you have to do it. Even if you miss a day, week, or year, it doesn't matter. Always focus on the positive and your enthusiasm will grow.

In Buddhism, discipline is seen as a mind delighting in virtue. The discipline of doing something on a regular basis is incredibly satisfying, will increase your ability to learn new moves, and will familiarize your mind and body with the principles and qualities present within tai chi much more than if you just practice once a week in a class. Without discipline, you cannot succeed at anything, but discipline need not be heavy and demanding—in fact, it can be the opposite.

Inertia (the state of the mind and body that results in laziness and following excuses) can prevent you from achieving your potential in any field and is usually the biggest factor keeping you from achieving what you want in life. If you want to achieve the benefits of tai chi, then overcoming inertia may be a factor. Enthusiasm is one of our most powerful allies. Don't give way to your excuses—practice with a happy mind. One of the hidden teachings of tai chi is to practice with the corners of the mouth turned upward. Try it.

finding a teacher

People often ask me to recommend a teacher or to explain to them how they can tell a good teacher from a bad one. Over the years, I have realized that there is no simple answer to this question. Finding a tai chi teacher is not hard, as most towns and cities now have a choice of teachers of varying styles, approaches, and abilities. However, finding a good teacher is not always easy—as anyone can open a tai chi class—so you need to rely on word of mouth, professional organizations, and your intuition and gut feelings. No one can really say what is right and wrong, but having visited classes of many teachers and heard many stories from my own students, I would recommend that when you search for a class, ask the teacher how long they have been practicing, who they have learned from, and whether they have any certification to teach.

It is, of course, possible to find a great teacher who doesn't hold a formal qualification; they may just have been allowed to teach by their own master or teacher. In most cases, a teacher should have at least four years of study behind them and have worked with an established teacher themselves. Any teacher who has learned tai chi in a weekend, or only from a book, should be avoided. Initially, though, it is best to find a competent teacher who knows what they are doing, but without a huge ego and the desire to make a lot of money from you!

tips on finding the right teacher for you

1. observe the quality of their movements.
Are their movements smooth, is their balance good, do their movements seem connected and flowing?

2. are they good at communicating?
To teach effectively, your teacher should be a skilled communicator, especially as the concepts behind tai chi are often complex or seem strange to the uninitiated.

3. is it a martial arts class or a self-help group?
Some classes have a more martial orientation than others, while some emphasize relaxation and healing. In some extreme cases tai chi classes offer group therapy, and much of the class may involve sharing feelings and emotions. Although this kind of work can be beneficial, it is not tai chi and is best avoided if advertised as such. If you are seeking group therapy, find an appropriately qualified therapist rather than a tai chi class.

Most tai chi classes do include an element of martial practice that can be helpful when understanding the movements and what they were originally used for. However, the majority of classes taught will emphasize de-stressing and self-healing, but you should also be aware that some tai chi classes can be very martially orientated, and if you are not expecting that, you may be in for a bit of a shock! Tai chi is a very broad art, so decide which end of the spectrum interests you most and check with the teacher as to the orientation of the class.

4. what is the "energy" of the class like?

The atmosphere of a class depends on what kind of person the teacher is, the venue in which they are teaching, and the people who attend. A good class should, in my opinion, be light, but with some seriousness, and the people attending it should be smiling at the end of the session, or at least looking more relaxed than they were when they stepped in. Above all, try to get a good perception of the class, the teacher, and the other people in the room. The atmosphere of the class is not determined only by whether it is "martial" or not. In my experience, some of the most respectful and kind teachers were also skilled fighters, and some of the biggest egoists are into self-healing (and vice versa).

5. does the teacher teach safely?

Teaching well includes making sure you are not injuring your students as you teach. Your teacher should be aware of the importance of body alignment and posture. Another important factor is whether the teacher is teaching material that is too advanced for you. Any teacher who claims to be able to teach you Taoist Alchemy or techniques for internal power in a weekend, or after a period of weeks, is best avoided. If it does not feel right to you, then it probably isn't. The only safe way to teach tai chi is to do so without forcing anything, which leads to a natural progresssion of ability.

Most tai chi classes include Chi Kung. Some Chi Kung exercises are very powerful, so powerful that they may, if practiced incorrectly, be dangerous to one's physical and mental health. The vast majority of Chi Kung exercises, however, are completely safe.

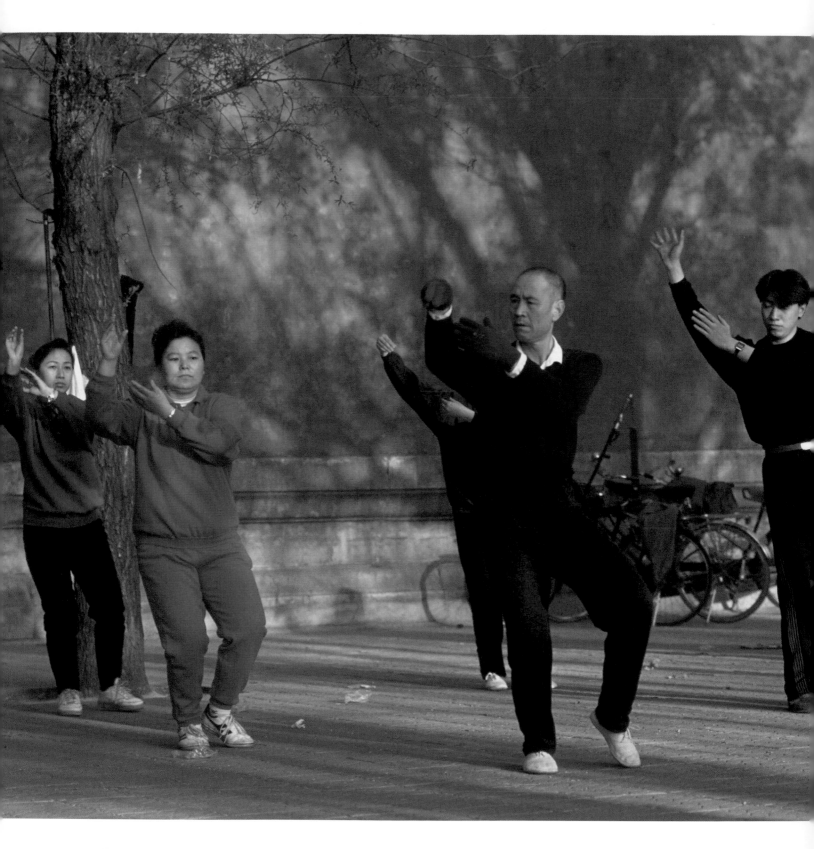

above: Practicing tai chi as a class or in a group can be extremely satisfying.

tai chi organizations

The Devon School of Tai Chi Chuan
For details of courses and for getting in touch with Matthew Rochford.
www.devontaichi.co.uk
e-mail: info@devontaichi.co.uk

The Wu Kung Federation
For seminars and teacher training with Peter Warr.
www.wu-kung-federation.co.uk
warrpeterwarr@aol.com

Taoist Tai Chi Society of the United States
1310 North Monroe Street
Tallahassee, FL 32303
tel: (850) 224-5438
e-mail: usa@ttcs.org

International Yang Style Tai Chi Chuan Association
4076 148th Avenue NE
Redmond, WA 98052
USA
tel: (425) 869-1185

Wu Style Tai Chi Chuan Academy, Toronto
427A Queen Street West, 3rd Floor
Toronto, Ontario M5V 2A5
Canada
tel: (416) 597-8426
www.wustyle.com

American Chen Style Tai Chi Association
2051 Hollywood Boulevard
Hollywood, FL 33020
www.americanchentaichi.com

Plum Blossom International Federation
925 Taraval Street
San Francisco, CA 94116
tel: (415) 665-2488
www.plumblossom.net

The American Tai Chuan-Tao Association
10523 117th Drive North
Largo, FL 33773
tel: (727) 319-8854
e-mail: sigungjohn@taichuantao.com

Boston Kung Fu Tai Chi Institute
361 Newbury Street
Boston, MA 02115
tel: (617) 262-0600
www.taichi.com

Gin Soon Tai Chi Chuan Federation U.S.A.
33 Harrison Avenue, 2nd Floor
Boston, MA 0211
tel: (617) 542-4442
www.gstaichi.org

internet resources

www.taichi-online.com
www.lowcountrytaichi.com
www.patiencetaichi.com
www.posturepage.com
www.taichiwebsite.com
www.taichido.com
www.thetaichisite.com
www.classicaltaichi.com

books

Step-By-Step Tai Chi *(Fireside, 1994)* by Lam Kam Chuen
Exercise program encapsulating the fundamentals of tai chi in an easy-to-use format.

Beginner's Tai Chi Chuan *(Unique Publications, 2000)* by Vincent Chu
Analyzes both the practical and philosophical aspects of tai chi.

The Complete Idiot's Guide to Tai Chi *(Macmillan Publishing Company, 1999)* by Bill Douglas and Richard Yennie
A step-by-step guide to the art of tai chi.

Beginning Tai Chi *(Charles E. Tuttle, 1994)* by Tri Thong Dang
Clear and concise information for tai chi beginners.

The Essential Movements of Tai Chi *(Paradigm Publications, 1996)*
by John Kotsias
All-encompassing book with clear, carefully illustrated instructions.

Teach Yourself Tai Chi *(McGraw-Hill/Contemporary Books)*
by Robert Parry
Comprehensive guide for tai chi beginners.

Thorsons Principles of Tai Chi *(Thorsons Publishing, 1999)*
by Paul Brecher
Explains the underlying principles of tai chi, thus helping to deepen
the understanding of the art beyond the practical.

The Essence of Tai Chi *(Shambhala Publications, 1995)*
by Waysun Liao
Pocket-size book offering insight into the philosophy and practice of
tai chi.

**Complete Tai Chi: The Definitive Guide to Physical and Emotional
Self-Improvement** *(Charles E. Tuttle, 1993)* by Alfred Huang
An in-depth book tracing the history and theory of tai chi; discusses
the forms as a healing technique.

The Authentic I Ching *(Newcastle Publishing Inc, 1987)*
by Henry Wei
Guide to this ancient form of divination and book of wisdom.

Cheng Tzu's Thirteen Treatises on Tai Chi Chuan *(North Atlantic
Books, 1985)* by Cheng Man Ching
Interpretation of classic tai chi text by leading master Cheng who took
tai chi to New York in the 1960s.

The Complete Book of Tai Chi Chuan *(Element Books Limited,
1996)* by Wong Kiew Kit
Comprehensive guide to all tai chi styles.

The Essential Tao *(Harper Collins, 1991)* by Thomas Cleary
Beautful translation of Taoist texts.

index